In Praise of *Health Promotion and Quality of Life*

"Finally, here is a text that draws together the disparate concepts of health promotion, quality of life, and social determinants of health. It is long overdue and will contribute to advancing the field. The introduction of quality of life into this volume represents a new conceptualization.

"There is very little written on the connection between quality of life and health promotion. The text could be used as a supplement to foundational health promotion courses, or could be used as a core text for graduate level health promotion courses with a quality of life or determinants of health perspective. With the prolific growth of schools of public health in Canada, I would anticipate that more such courses are being developed, so the market is beginning to expand greatly."

— *Kim Raine, Centre for Health Promotion Studies, School of Public Health, University of Alberta*

"The book is an urgently needed compilation of critical perspectives on health promotion in Canada. I very much like the emphasis on how population health is intimately linked to the social determinants and the policy-related causes-of-the-causes. The book will make quite a splash in the somewhat stagnant waters of many current health promotion writings and teachings.

"The linkage between quality of life and public policy will be of great interest to the growing number of courses and programs in Canada that bring 'policy' and 'health' together. It has strong potential to be the same kind of catalytic book that Dr. Raphael's *Social Determinants of Health* has proven to be.

"The logical flow of the book makes very good intuitive sense ... In summary, the individual chapters are excellent stand-alone articles.

This means that the quality of the book is also superlative. This book is a testament to this editor's longstanding commitment to advancing scholarly work in Canada for the explicit purpose of progressive social change.

"For readers who are not overly familiar with the critical health literature, the links among these articles would be difficult to make without this book. So, the book will provide an important way for these readers to connect the dots. That being said, the book is very relevant for all who concern themselves with moving a social change agenda forward in Canada."

— *Elizabeth McGibbon, School of Nursing, St. Francis Xavier University*

"This book addresses a very significant issue in Canadian health promotion. I particularly appreciate the public policy focus and the emphasis on a broad conceptualization of quality of life. The articles are well written, making the work easily accessible to a variety of audiences, including students, practitioners, and researchers. This reader will encourage a broader view of the impact of health determinants on quality of life as experienced in day to day living."

— *Linda Reutter, Faculty of Nursing, University of Alberta*

HEALTH PROMOTION AND QUALITY OF LIFE IN CANADA

Essential Readings
Edited by Dennis Raphael

Health Promotion and Quality of Life in Canada
Edited by Dennis Raphael
First published in 2010 by Canadian Scholars' Press Inc.
180 Bloor Street West, Suite 801
Toronto, Ontario
M5S 2V6
www.cspi.org

The contributions in this volume—apart from the opening and concluding chapters—
are adaptations of previously published material.

Canadian Scholars' Press Inc./Women's Press gratefully acknowledges financial
support for our publishing activities from the Government of Canada through the
Book Publishing Industry Development Program (BPIDP), and the Government of
Ontario through the Ontario Book Publishing Tax Credit Program.

Library and Archives Canada Cataloguing in Publication
Health promotion and quality of life in Canada : essential readings / edited by
Dennis Raphael.

ISBN 978-1-55130-367-3
1. Health promotion— Canada . 2. Quality of life— Canada . 3. Medical
policy— Canada . 4. Public health—Social aspects— Canada .
I. Raphael, Dennis
RA418.3.C3H435 2010   362.10971   C2009-906640-8

Cover and typesetting design by Aldo Fierro

09 10 11 12 13   5 4 3 2 1

Printed and bound in Canada by Marquis Book Printing, Inc.

Table of Contents

Preface

During the late 1990s, Prime Minister Jean Chrétien constantly reminded Canadians that the United Nations Human Development Report (UNHDR) rated Canada first in "quality of life" using the Human Development Index. For many Canadians, however, such reveling seemed at odds with evidence of increasing financial, housing, and food insecurity among significant proportions of the population. (The UNHDR ranked Canada ninth for dealing with human and income poverty.) It was during this time that a team of researchers at the University of Toronto's Centre for Health Promotion began to specify the dimensions of quality of life using a health promotion framework.

The thrust of this work was an analysis of quality of life that not only placed the concept within a psychological, social, and community context, but also showed how the dynamic field of health promotion could provide a means of both explaining variations in quality of life and pointing the way towards improving it. The result was a series of increasingly complex analyses that considered quality of life as being firstly an individual issue, secondly a community issue, and ultimately a societal issue. The work was then able to draw upon the emerging concern with the social determinants of health to show how social determinants such as income, employment security and working conditions, food, housing, and education were important contributors to quality of life as well as being determinants of health.

But what were the determinants of the determinants? How was it that increasing numbers of Canadians were coming to experience income, employment, housing, and food security? Why was the quality of the social determinants of health in Canada coming to be so different than their quality in other nations? The answer seemed to lie in variations in public policy concerned with the distribution of material and social resources amongst the population. The antecedents of these public policies appeared to have a lot to do with the form the welfare state was taking in these differing jurisdictions. And there were clear political and ideological components to these differing forms of the welfare state. The contributions to this volume trace the development of quality of life from the initial concern with specifying the components of individual quality of life right up to the political and economic analysis of national approaches to welfare provision.

The first section of the book provides a conceptual basis for determining whether an individual or community is achieving a good quality of life. It provides the components of a model of quality of life with wide applicability across populations and levels of society. The model of quality of life is related to principles of health promotion that have proven to be influential in shaping health promotion research and practice in Canada and elsewhere.

The second section of the book shows how quality of life is related to community structures and public policies that determine how material and other resources are distributed amongst societal members. It provides reports of community quality of life and public policy studies—with information provided by community members themselves—that show how quality of life is related to public policy decisions made by governments. These public policy decisions appear to be influenced by the shape and quality of a nation's welfare state.

The third section of the book draws upon recent work on the social determinants of health to place quality of life within a political economy framework. It uses the social determinants concept to show how nations differ in how willing they are to support the quality of life and health of their members. Recent work is summarized and key issues identified. Within this framework, Canada does not do well as compared to other nations. These broader concepts are consistent with principles of health promotion as articulated by the World Health Organization.

The fourth section focuses on the quality of life situations of four vulnerable groups in Canadian society: Aboriginal populations, immigrants and persons of colour, persons with disabilities, and women. Each of these groups experiences both poorer quality of life and exposures to poorer social determinants of health than white males of European descent. These groups have also been the focus of concerted health promotion and public policy advocacy.

The fifth section suggests means by which a quality of life agenda focused on improving public policymaking can be advanced. After identifying the profound barriers to having such an agenda moving forward, various avenues of academic inquiry and citizen activity are suggested. Increasing concern with quality of life by various governmental and non-governmental institutions is seen as supporting such an ambitious agenda. There is a special role for the health sector to play in these activities, but to date such activity has been limited.

It is hoped that the reader will experience the same kind of transformation in thinking about quality of life as did the working group at the Centre for Health Promotion. In the end, promoting quality of life requires action at all levels: the individual, the community, and the societal. To date, the focus on the individual—and their quality of life—by most academic disciplines and helping professions has led to a profound neglect of the community and societal. Hopefully, this volume will serve to help correct this imbalance. And, by the way, in 2007 Canada had lost its first-place ranking and was now ranked fourth in the Human Development Index and twelfth in human and income poverty by the United Nations.

Dennis Raphael
October 1, 2009

Introduction

CHAPTER 1

Setting the Stage: Why Quality of Life? Why Health Promotion?

Dennis Raphael

> It shall be lawful for the Queen, by and with the Advice and
> Consent of the Senate and House of Commons, to make
> Laws for the Peace, Order, and good Government of Canada.
> (Government of Canada, 1867/1982)

INTRODUCTION

During the first decade of the 21st century, Canada faces a variety of threats to one of its founding concepts, that of *Peace, Order, and good Government.* Income and wealth inequality are growing and Canadian poverty levels remain amongst the highest of wealthy developed nations (Organisation for Economic Co-operation and Development, 2008). Democratic participation in the form of voter levels and political activities is declining and many Canadians express concern about the future (Canadian Policy Research Networks, 2002). Increasingly, Canadians feel that governments and other major societal institutions are not responsive to their voices and needs.

Despite increasing life expectancy and declines in mortality rates from some of the major killers such as heart disease and cancers, Canada's relative national ranking on many indicators of health status as compared to other wealthy developed nations is either stagnating or declining (Organisation for Economic Co-operation and Development, 2007). As one example, during the time period 1980

1

to 2002 Canada's relative ranking on a key indicator of population health—the infant mortality rate—slipped from 10th to 23rd (Robert Wood Johnson Foundation, 2008). As another example, Canada performs relatively poorly on numerous indicators of children's health and well-being such as death by injury and the teenage pregnancy rate (Innocenti Research Centre, 2001).

Furthermore, a recent report that examined Canadian children's performance on numerous indicators of well-being provided Canada with an overall ranking of 12th of 21 wealthy developed nations (Innocenti Research Centre, 2007). More specifically, Canada's thematic rankings were as follows: material well-being, sixth of 21; health and safety, 13th; family and peer relationships, 18th; behaviours and risks, 17th; and subjective well-being, 15th. Only in educational well-being did Canada do very well (second).

There is ample reason to believe that these troubling indicators result in large part from Canadian governmental authorities' unwillingness to address a series of emerging issues. One such issue, the incidence of poverty, finds Canada performing very poorly in comparison with other wealthy developed nations (Organisation for Economic Co-operation and Development, 2008). Canada's ranking for incidence of poverty for adults (with first = lowest rate of poverty and 30th = highest rate of poverty) is 19th among the wealthy industrialized nations of the Organisation for Economic Co-operation and Development; for families with children, Canada ranks 21st; and for rates of child poverty, 20th. Canada's investment of national wealth in public spending on early childhood education and care, education, families, seniors, persons with disabilities, and employment support and training is among the lowest of wealthy developed nations (Raphael, 2007a).

Numerous indicators of Canada's social safety net—for example, unemployment benefits, social assistance rates, and levels of minimum wages—provide a similar picture: Canada's provision of various forms of security and supports to citizens is meagre as compared to many other wealthy developed nations (Raphael, 2007a). There is a clear emerging consensus that Canada's approach towards citizen provision is problematic and related to a variety of societal ills (Raphael, 2007b). Increasingly, Canadians are looking for means of identifying these concerns and responding to these issues. All of these issues are about quality of life.

Improving quality of life can take many forms. Clinical health care, psychology, social work, and public health services can respond to individuals who manifest adverse reactions to individual, community, and societal conditions—for example, illness, distress, hunger, isolation, and adoption of risk behaviours—one patient or client at a time. The health care and social assistance systems are based upon such an approach. Community development activities can facilitate community members coming together to identify and address local concerns and formulate appropriate responses. Many community organizations and agencies apply this concept in an attempt to engage citizens in addressing issues and bringing them to the attention of governmental and agency authorities.

The political arena provides yet another realm in which concerned citizens can act to address quality of life issues. Issue-related social movements—for example, advocates for improved housing, childcare, employment conditions, health care, food security, income security, anti-racism, women's issues, and community safety—strive to raise their issues with either governing or opposition political parties. Their goal is to have these issues addressed through governmental action.

Although concern about the vitality of Canada's democratic structures is growing, Canada's political parties represent a diversity of views on numerous societal issues and provide institutions by which citizens can be engaged with the political process, if they wish to be so. Such diversity of opinion ranging from conservative to social democratic is not seen in the USA, where the two main political parties are rather conservative in comparison to those of other wealthy developed nations. The USA does not have a viable social democratic party (Lipset & Marks, 2000).

The rationale for this volume is that the concepts of quality of life and health promotion can help define and provide means of addressing emerging Canadian concerns. *Quality of life* is a multidimensional concept that allows consideration of a range of perspectives from individual subjective well-being through to broader indicators of societal functioning. Quality of life has meaning and relevance for the average person and incorporates perspectives from disciplines such as disabilities, economics, health studies, medicine, psychology, sociology, social work, and political science, among others.

Health promotion provides a framework within which Canadians—both lay and professional—can address these issues (O'Neill, Pederson, Dupéré, & Rootman, 2007). Its approach to encouraging citizen engagement in the service of improving the determinants of health and well-being is ideally suited for improving quality of life. Quality of life and health promotion as approaches to addressing societal issues are especially relevant to Canada because many quality of life and health promotion concepts originated here (Raphael, 2008a).

WHY QUALITY OF LIFE?

> . There is no single best set of outcomes or indicators for mea-
> suring quality of life issues, but parliamentarians should
> strive to create fair, open, transparent and inclusive mea-
> sures that respond to citizen needs and wishes. (Bennett,
> Lenihan, Williams, & Young, 2001, p. 10)

Quality of life is a concept that has meaning for citizens, professionals, and governmental authorities. Much of this has to do with its intuitive or common sense notion of it representing "the good life." The average person may not know exactly what quality of life is, but does seem to know whether their own quality of life is good or bad. Quality of life is also a concept that has been taken up by many professionals as indicating whether their treatments and services result in either good or bad outcomes. And it is increasingly common for governmental authorities to assure citizens that their policymaking is concerned with improving citizens' quality of life. Much activity has gone into developing quality of life approaches for each of these uses. The papers contained in this volume detail these approaches.

Quality of life is a *normative* concept. What this means is that there are clear expectations of what quality of life should be. Quality of life of individuals, communities, and societies should be good, not bad. And if it is not good then something needs to be done to improve it. This seems rather obvious, but much academic research in quality-of-life-related areas acts as if there is no place for judgments or value statements on the parts of theory builders and researchers. This latter approach, also known as positive or objective science, reflects a reluctance to identify issues as being particularly problematic for the health and well-being of citizens and a reluctance to make recommendations for policy action on the part of governments (Raphael, Curry-Stevens, & Bryant, 2008).

Quality of life can therefore be considered as a desired quality of individuals, communities, or even societies. Numerous models of such a state exist, and the ones favoured in this volume are the quality of life model developed at the University of Toronto and the social determinants of health approach developed at York University.

Actual quality of life assessments can be based on a variety of forms of data. These include objective (e.g., quantitative, survey, and statistical) and subjective (e.g., qualitative, interview, and thematic) assessments; individual and community-sited data gathering (e.g., characteristics of individuals or features of communities); and the application of a range of broadly defined societal indicators (e.g., societal poverty rates, governmental service provision, and population health status). Quality of life assessment can therefore range from considering elements of broad societal indicators to the actual lived experience of individual persons. All of these approaches are valuable for considering quality of life and what needs to be done to improve it.

Quality of life of individuals, communities, and societies can be placed within a public policy perspective. While individual, family, and community characteristics and features and specific aspects of medical treatments and social services received by individuals and communities certainly influence quality of life, public policies developed by governing authorities have profound effects upon quality of life. As one example, Canada's lack of any recognizable early childhood education and care system has significant effects upon the quality of life of children, families, and especially women (Friendly, 2008). As another, Canada's relatively high family poverty rate has strong implications for the quality of life of both families living in poverty and the rest of society (Raphael, 2007c). The quality of Canada's social safety net also contributes to quality of life, especially for the most disadvantaged. The implications of public policymaking form the basis for much of the content of this volume.

Finally, quality of life—however defined—is influenced by a variety of economic, political, and social forces that differ systematically among nations. What is it about nations whose quality of life seems to be so superior to quality of life in other nations? Is there something about the operation of their economic and political systems that creates public policies that support quality of life? If so, how can the practices of these nations be incorporated into Canadian public policymaking in the service of strengthening quality of life?

Among many quality of life researchers, there is a reluctance to consider how the political ideologies of governing authorities contribute to the presence of quality of life issues. There is also a reluctance to identify political solutions (i.e., how policymaking and implementation on the parts of governing authorities) could respond to these problems. Avoidance of the political is common to many academic disciplines such as education, health sciences, psychology, and sociology, among others. These issues, however, are addressed in this volume.

WHY HEALTH PROMOTION?

> Health promotion is the process of enabling people to increase control over, and to improve, their health. (WHO, 1986)

The role Canada has played in the development and application of health promotion is well documented in *Health Promotion: An Anthology* (Restrepo, 2000), *Health Promotion in Canada: Provincial, National, and International Perspectives* (Pederson, O'Neill, & Rootman, 1994), and *Health Promotion in Canada: Critical Perspectives* (O'Neill et al., 2007). Table 1.1 provides some key events. Recent reviews of health promotion in Canada are also available (Poland, 2007; Raphael, 2008a).

Table 1.1: Key Developments in Health Promotion in Canada

1974	Lalonde Report
1980	Shifting Medical Paradigm Conference
1984	Beyond Health Care Conference
1986	The Ottawa Charter
1986	The Epp Report
1994	Federal/Provincial/Territorial Report on Population Health
1994	Publication of *Why Are Some People Healthy and Others Not?*
2000	Health Canada Population Health Template
2002	Social Determinants of Health Across the Life-Span Conference
2008	Chief Public Health Officer of Canada's Report on the State of Public Health in Canada

Sources: Labonte, 1994; Legowski & McKay, 2000; O'Neill, et al., 2007; Raphael, 2008c.

Health promotion provides a framework for efforts to improve the quality of life of individuals, communities, and societies by applying a wide range of activities and approaches to achieve desired outcomes. It is also about citizen engagement, an important part of how democratic processes can improve quality of life. The most succinct statements of the principles and values of health promotion are contained in the Ottawa Charter for Health Promotion, which was presented at the first International Conference on Health Promotion: "Health promotion is the process of enabling people to increase control over, and to improve, their health" (World Health Organization, 1986). In line with its predominantly societal approach to promoting health, the Charter outlines the basic *prerequisites for health* as being peace, shelter, education, food, income, a stable ecosystem, sustainable resources, social justice, and equity.

Health promotion, as outlined in the Charter and subsequent World Health Organization statements, is based on a commitment to improving health and well-being through five pillars of action: building healthy public policy; creating supportive environments; strengthening community action; developing personal skills; and reorienting health services.

The Action Statement for Health Promotion in Canada represents the high-water mark in health-promoting thinking in Canada (Canadian Public Health Association, 1996). It identifies advocating for healthy public policies as the single best strategy to affect the determinants of health. Priority areas include reducing inequalities in income and wealth; strengthening communities through local alliances to change unhealthy living conditions; supporting environments that promote healthy lifestyles; and developing a settings approach to practice. Community development is also a priority.

The most well-developed policy-oriented approach to promoting health and well-being, the Healthy Cities Movement, originated in Canada but has come to fruition in Europe (World Health Organization Regional Office for Europe, 2003). Healthy Cities promotes innovation and change in local health policy, advocating new approaches to public health. But the movement also makes explicit some key issues germane to both health promotion and improving quality of life. Healthy Cities projects are said to have six key characteristics.

1. *Commitment to health:* They are based upon a commitment to health. They affirm the holistic nature of health, recognizing the interaction between its physical, mental, social, and spiritual dimensions. Promotion of health and prevention of disease are their priorities. Health can be created through the cooperative efforts of individuals and groups in the city.

2. *Political decision-making:* Projects require political decision-making for public health. Housing, environment, education, social services, and other programs of city government have a major effect on the state of health in cities. Healthy Cities projects strengthen the contribution of such programs to health by influencing the political decisions of city councils.

3. *Intersectoral action:* They generate intersectoral action by which organizations working outside the health sector can contribute more to health. Healthy Cities projects create organizational mechanisms through which city departments and other bodies come together to negotiate their contribution to such action.

4. *Community participation:* Projects emphasize community participation. People participate in health through their lifestyle choices, their use of health services, their views on health issues, and their work in community groups. Healthy Cities projects promote more active roles for people in all of these areas. People can have a direct influence on project decisions and the activities of city departments and other organizations.

5. *Innovation:* They work through processes of innovation. Promoting health and preventing disease through intersectoral action requires a constant search for new ideas and methods. Healthy Cities projects create opportunities for innovation within a climate that supports change. They spread knowledge of innovative methods, create incentives for innovation, and recognize the achievements of those who experiment with new policies and programs.

6. *Healthy public policy:* Their outcome is healthy public policy. Healthy Cities create settings for health throughout the city administration. Projects achieve their goals when homes, schools, workplaces, and other parts of the urban environment become healthier settings in which to live. Political decisions, intersectoral action, community participation, and innovation promoted through Healthy Cities projects work together to achieve healthy public policy.

The Belfast Declaration provides the latest thinking concerning the Healthy Cities approach (World Health Organization, 2003). The declaration emphasizes the importance of partnerships at all levels and of good governance. Specific areas of action include reducing inequalities and addressing poverty; assessing the health impacts of policy decisions; and taking an active role in shaping and implementing strategies for health. Since cities cannot act alone, national governments must recognize that national policies on health have a local dimension and acknowledge the importance of cities.

Any activity concerned with improving quality of life—whether an explicit "health promotion" activity or not—can benefit from incorporating the six principles of the Healthy Cities approach. As just one example of the power of such an approach, consider the emerging concern with what are termed the social determinants of health.

SOCIAL DETERMINANTS OF HEALTH, HEALTH PROMOTION, AND QUALITY OF LIFE

Internationally, the World Health Organization's establishment of an International Commission on the Social Determinants of Health has stimulated discussion on the societal factors that shape health and well-being. The final report of the commission is now available, as are numerous final reports dealing with a range of important issues (Commission on the Social Determinants of Health, 2008). Two of the commission's knowledge networks (Globalization and Health and Early Childhood Development) were centred in Canada, and another (Workplace Health) had significant Canadian representation. The concept has enjoyed increased mention in the international academic literature and reviews are available (Graham, 2004, 2007; Raphael, 2008c). The Canadian Senate's Subcommittee on Population Health has undertaken a review of the social determinants of health (Senate Subcommittee on Population Health, 2008).

The social determinants of health concept is concerned with how the organization of societies shapes health and well-being (Raphael, 2008b). Social determinants of health have been defined as the economic and social conditions that shape the health of individuals, communities, and jurisdictions as a whole. The concept shows many similarities with the prerequisites of health contained in the Ottawa Charter for Health Promotion. A variety of contemporary approaches to social determinants of health are available but, in this volume, social determinants of health refers to Aboriginal status, early life, education, employment and working conditions, food security, gender, health care services, housing, income and its distribution, social safety net, social exclusion and unemployment and employment security.

The implications of the social determinants of health for quality of life and health promotion issues are obvious. Social determinants are probably as strong determinants of quality of life as they are of health. And social determinants of health are also profoundly influenced by public policy and can therefore be the targets of health promotion activity. Can the increasing concern with quality of life and the social determinants of health be applied in the service of health promotion? Fran Baum, a member of the International Commission on the Social Determinants of Health argues:

> As the challenges confronting us in the twenty-first century grow ... health promotion needs a new bible that equips it to contribute to these challenges. The Commission on the Social Determinants of Health's final report provides such a document by providing a global overview of the importance of the social determinants of health and the centrality of privileging strategies that create fairness both between and within countries ... The health promotion movement has the possibility of re-inventing itself in the twenty-first century to offer the holistic understanding of health, the skills, passion and commitment required to be the core of a social movement which advocates for new healthy, equitable and sustainable economic and social structures globally and within countries. (Baum, 2008, p. 464)

CONCLUSION

Good quality of life is a desired goal for individuals, communities, and societies. There is evidence that on any number of indicators of quality of life, Canada does not fare as well as many other wealthy developed nations. There are a variety of models by which quality of life can be considered and various means by which it can be assessed. There are a number of ways by which quality of life can be improved. Individual service delivery can improve quality of life as can community development and the development of healthy public policy. Such activities may also require activity in the political realm.

In this volume, the implications of a health promotion approach for improving quality of life are explored. Aspects of health promotion that appear particularly relevant for this effort include the importance of engaging citizens in policy-related activity in the service of influencing the determinants of health. The recent concern with how various aspects of society shape health—the social determinants of health—can help inform these efforts. Social determinants of health are also strong determinants of quality of life. And social determinants of health are themselves shaped by public policymaking, thereby making them a target of health promotion activity. How these differing perspectives can come together in the service of improving quality of life forms the basis of this collection.

REFERENCES

Baum, F. (2008). The Commission on the Social Determinants of Health: Reinventing health promotion for the twenty-first century? *Critical Public Health, 18*(4), 457–466.

Bennett, C., Lenihan, D., Williams, J., & Young, W. (2001). *Measuring quality of life: The use of societal outcomes by parliamentarians. Changing government* (Vol. 3). Ottawa, ON: Library of Congress.

Canadian Policy Research Networks. (2002). *Quality of life in Canada: A citizens' report card.* Retrieved June 23, 2008, from www.cprn.org/doc.cfm?doc=44&l=en

Canadian Public Health Association. (1996). *Action statement for health promotion in Canada.* Retrieved June 23, 2008, from http://www.cpha.ca/en/programs/policy/action.aspx. Ottawa, ON. Canadian Public Health Association.

Commission on the Social Determinants of Health. (2008). *Closing the gap in a generation: Health equity through action on the social determinants of health.* Geneva: World Health Organization.

Friendly, M. (2008). Early childhood education and care as a social determinant of health. In D. Raphael (Ed.), *Social determinants of health: Canadian perspectives* (2nd ed., pp. 128–142). Toronto, ON: Canadian Scholars' Press Inc.

Government of Canada. (1867/1982). *The Constitution Act, 1867*. Retrieved June 23, 2008, from http://laws.justice.gc.ca/en/const/c1867_e.html

Graham, H. (2004). Social determinants and their unequal distribution: Clarifying policy understandings. *Milbank Quarterly, 82*(1), 101–124.

Graham, H. (2007). *Unequal lives: Health and socioeconomic inequalities*. New York: Open University Press.

Innocenti Research Centre. (2001). *A league table of teenage births in rich nations*. Florence: Innocenti Research Centre.

Innocenti Research Centre. (2007). *An overview of child well-being in rich countries: A comprehensive assessment of the lives and well-being of children and adolescents in the economically advanced nations*. Florence: Innocenti Research Centre.

Labonte, R. (1994). Death of a program: Birth of a metaphor. Health promotion in Canada: Provincial, national and international perspectives. In I. Rootman, A. Pederson, & M. O'Neill (eds.), *Health promotion in Canada: Provincial national and international perspectives*, pp. 72–90. Toronto, ON: WB Saunders.

Legowski, B., & L. McKay (2000). *Health beyond health care: Twenty-five years of federal health policy development*. Ottawa, ON: Canadian Policy Research Networks.

Lipset, M., & Marks, G. (2000). *It didn't happen here: Why socialism failed in the United States*. New York: WW Norton.

O'Neill, M., Pederson, A., Dupéré, S., & Rootman, I. (Eds.). (2007). *Health promotion in Canada: Critical perspectives*. Toronto, ON: Canadian Scholars' Press Inc.

Organisation for Economic Co-operation and Development. (2007). *Health at a glance 2007, OECD indicators*. Paris: Organisation for Economic Co-operation and Development.

Organisation for Economic Co-operation and Development. (2008). *Growing unequal? Income distribution and poverty in OECD nations*. Paris: Organisation for Economic Co-operation and Development.

Pederson, A., O'Neill, M., & Rootman, I. (1994). *Health promotion in Canada: Provincial, national, and international perspectives*. Toronto, ON: WB Saunders.

Poland, B. (2007). Health promotion in Canada: Perspectives and future prospects. *Revista Brasileira em Promoção da Saúde, 20*(1), 3–11.

Raphael, D. (2007a). Canadian public policy and poverty in international perspective. In D. Raphael (Ed.), *Poverty and policy in Canada: Implications for health and quality of life* (pp. 335–364). Toronto, ON: Canadian Scholars' Press Inc.

Raphael, D. (2007b). The future of the Canadian welfare state. In D. Raphael (Ed.), *Poverty and policy in Canada: Implications for health and quality of life* (pp. 365-398). Toronto, ON: Canadian Scholars' Press Inc.

Raphael, D. (2007c). *Poverty and policy in Canada: Implications for health and quality of life.* Toronto, ON: Canadian Scholars' Press Inc.

Raphael, D. (2008a). Grasping at straws: A recent history of health promotion in Canada. *Critical Public Health, 18*(4), 483-495.

Raphael, D. (2008b). Introduction to the social determinants of health. In D. Raphael (Ed.), *Social determinants of health: Canadian perspectives* (2nd ed., pp. 2-19). Toronto, ON: Canadian Scholars' Press Inc.

Raphael, D. (Ed.). (2008c). *Social determinants of health: Canadian perspectives* (2nd ed.). Toronto, ON: Canadian Scholars' Press Inc.

Raphael, D., Curry-Stevens, A., & Bryant, T. (2008). Barriers to addressing the social determinants of health: Insights from the Canadian experience. *Health Policy, 88,* 222-235.

Restrepo, H. E. (2000). *Health promotion: An anthology.* Washington, DC: Pan American Health Organization.

Robert Wood Johnson Foundation. (2008). *Overcoming obstacles to health.* Princeton, NJ: Robert Wood Johnson Foundation.

Senate Subcommittee on Population Health. (2008). *Canada Senate Subcommittee reports: International community's approach to population health.* Retrieved March 15, 2008, from http://health-equity.blogspot.com/2008/03/eq-canada-senate-subcommittee-reports.html

World Health Organization. (1986). *Ottawa charter for health promotion, 1986.* Retrieved June 23, 2009, from www.euro.who.int/AboutWHO/Policy/20010827_2

World Health Organization. (2003). *Belfast declaration for healthy cities.* Retrieved June 23, 2009, from http://www.euro.who.int/document/Hcp/Belfast_DEC_E.pdf

World Health Organization Regional Office for Europe. (2003). *Healthy cities: Books and published technical documents.* Retrieved March 15, 2008, from www.euro.who.int/healthy-cities/publications/20030206_3

Part I: Individual Perspectives

Part I is an introduction to the concept of quality of life (QOL) and how it has been applied in numerous health-related areas. The focus is upon the QOL model developed by the Centre for Health Promotion at the University of Toronto. The theoretical background to the model is presented and two individual-level applications are described.

Chapter 2 provides an overview of various approaches to considering QOL. These range from very medically oriented approaches, where the primary focus is upon individual patients and their responses to specific medical treatments, right through to analyses of the manner in which societies are acting to meet the needs of citizens. The contributions of two QOL approaches that are influenced by World Health Organization concepts of health are highlighted.

Chapter 3 provides an elaboration of the QOL model developed by the Centre for Health Promotion at the University of Toronto. Details concerning the model's conceptual basis, the manner of its development, and its application to analysis of the QOL of persons with developmental disabilities are highlighted. The implications of QOL assessments for a variety of health promotion applications are provided.

In Chapters 4 and 5, specific applications of the Centre for Health Promotion QOL model, as applied to individuals, are presented. The development of these instruments was based on the QOL model and its items grounded in the views and perceptions of the group for which it was developed. Chapter 4 details the development and validation of the QOL Profile—Adolescent Version, while Chapter 5 does the same for the QOL Profile—Seniors Version. These instruments are shown to be both reliable and valid, and suggested applications are presented.

CHAPTER 2

Quality of Life Indicators and Health

Dennis Raphael, Rebecca Renwick, Ivan Brown, and Irving Rootman

OVERVIEW AND PURPOSE

Quality of life considerations are increasingly influencing the planning, delivery, and evaluation of social, health, and medical services (Parmenter, 1994; Renwick et al., 1996). That is, improved quality of life is seen as a desired outcome of service provision. Quality of life assessments can also identify individuals at risk for poor health outcomes even in the absence of diagnosable illness or other problems (Raphael et al., 1994). Within these health promotion and illness prevention perspectives, quality of life issues inform interventions that contribute to health by modifying environments. Quality of life is also an important issue in the disabilities area where at least four recent volumes have appeared (Brown et al., 1992; Goode, 1994; Romney et al., 1994; Schalock, 1990a).

The increasing emphasis upon quality of life in the health and related disability and rehabilitation literatures continues primarily within a tradition of emphasizing illness and disability, rather than health and ability. That is, health is seen primarily as the absence of illness or disability rather than a resource for daily living. Similarly, most approaches espouse an individually oriented micro-level perspective, rather than a system or macro-level perspective. In this article, we review current quality of life perspectives in relation to health status and health promotion. We then consider two emerging quality of life models that provide a heuristic for expanding the range of inquiry into the relationship between quality of life and health.

DEFINING QUALITY OF LIFE

Though concern with quality of life has been an important human concern since antiquity, social science research into the concept gained prominence following Thorndike's (1939) work on life in cities. Despite its long history in the literature, though, there is disagreement on how quality of life should be defined and measured, a state of affairs common within a variety of fields (see Naess, 1987).

ISSUES IN MEASURING QUALITY OF LIFE

Issues in measuring quality of life are similar to those found in social science research methodology debates. In this paper we consider four main issues. A first issue is whether the focus should be on objective indicators (e.g., medical status, mobility, quality of housing) or subjective indicators of satisfaction (e.g., satisfaction with health, mobility, housing). A second issue is whether data should describe and be collected from individuals (micro-level data, either objective or subjective, possibly aggregated up to population units) or describe the functioning of systems (e.g., income distribution, availability of health services). A third question is whether measures should be explicitly value-laden (e.g., personal control and independence are fundamental quality of life indicators) or value-neutral (e.g., personal control and independence may be desirable for only some individuals). Fourth, an issue that is most apparent in the discussion of social indicator models is whether measures should be closely related to social policy and social change goals.

HEALTH-RELATED QUALITY OF LIFE

In the health sciences area, quality of life has traditionally been used as an outcome variable to evaluate the effectiveness of medical treatments (Hollandsworth, 1988) and rehabilitation efforts (Livneh, 1988).

Health-Related Quality of Life: Medical Approaches

Spilker's (1990) approach to quality of life illustrates the emerging medical view. He suggests assessing quality of life through examination of four domains: (1) physical status and functional abilities; (2) psychological status and well-being; (3) social interactions; and (4) economic status and economic factors. These include both objective and subjective assessments. Additionally, he highlights the importance of having the patient provide an overall subjective assessment of quality of life, described as "an individual's overall satisfaction with life, and one's general sense of personal well-being" (p. 4).

Schipper, Clinch, and Powell's (1990) definition of quality of life is therefore closely linked to the effects of illness upon individuals and the measurement of day-to-day competencies and abilities:

> Quality of life represents the functional effect of an illness and it's consequent therapy upon a patient, as perceived by the patient. Four broad domains contribute to the overall effect: physical and occupational function; psychologic state; social interaction; and somatic sensation. This definition is based upon the premise that the goal of medicine is to make the morbidity and mortality of a particular disease disappear. We seek to take away the disease and its consequences, and leave the patient as if untouched by the illness. (p. 16)

The medical approach is clear in relation to the four quality of life issues. There is an orientation towards objective indicators of functioning at the individual level. The subjective report of the individual is gaining increasing importance however. Discussion concerning issues of the role of values in developing measures of quality of life and the relationship of measures to social policy or social change is virtually non-existent.

Health-Related Quality of Life: Health-Oriented Approaches

Recently, a more health-related, rather than illness-related, literature on quality of life has appeared. Some attempt is made to focus upon health rather than illness, and positive rather than negative aspects of behavioural functioning. Bowling's (1991) review of traditional measures of health outcomes highlights the customary reliance upon mortality, morbidity, service utilization, and subjective reports of illness. Many of the indices found in *Measuring Health: A Review of Quality of Life Instruments* (Bowling, 1991), as well as McDowell and Newell's (1987) *Measuring Health*, focus on disability and illness-related aspects of functioning.

As Bowling points out, it is only when one takes seriously the World Health Organization (WHO) definition of health as involving physical, mental, and social well-being, and not merely the absence of disease or infirmity, does focus upon indices of positive physical, mental, and social well-being occur. Nevertheless, similar to those working within medically oriented quality of life, those focusing upon concepts of health and wellness often define quality of life by emphasizing the effects of illness:

> Basically, quality of life is recognized as a concept representing individual responses to the physical, mental, and social effects of illness on daily living which influence the extent to which personal satisfaction with life circumstances can be achieved. (Bowling, 1991, p. 9)

The *Medical Outcomes Study* (Stewart and Ware, 1992) illustrates a large-scale application of the health-related quality of life approach to a variety of medical conditions.

The health-related approach is oriented towards both objective and subjective indicators of functioning. Focus is primarily at the individual level and discussion concerning issues of the role of values, in this case the WHO definition of health, is acknowledged. A link between quality of life measures and work related to social policy or social change models is uncommon.

THE SOCIAL DIAGNOSIS APPROACH

In Green and Kreuter's (1991) model of health promotion, assessing quality of life concerns is part of the social diagnosis phase of program development. They argue that health outcomes are embedded in the broader life concerns encompassed by quality of life. Thus, the community's concerns about quality of life provide the context for understanding how health-related issues could be raised within communities by health promoters.

The health promoter, by understanding the quality of life concerns of the community, demonstrates for the community the connections between their quality of life concerns and health issues. Green and Kreuter's contribution to the quality of life discussion is to highlight the need to bring the community into the development, implementation, and evaluation of health services and promotion programs. The methods by which a social diagnosis is carried out involve community-oriented applied methods, such as focus groups, community forums, and community surveys. However, Green and Kreuter fail to define quality of life. They simply allude to some possibilities and outline means of assessing quality of life, whatever it may be:

> The term, quality of life, like the concepts of health and love, is difficult to define and still more difficult to measure. Nevertheless, many approaches are available for assessing the quality of life in communities, both objectively and subjectively. Objective measures include social indicators, such as unemployment rates, and descriptions of such environmental features as housing density and air quality. More critical to the educational approach are subjective assessments, using information from the community members as a primary indicator of quality of life concerns. In this approach the adjustment and life satisfaction of community members are surveyed. (p. 48)

The social diagnosis approach emphasizes subjective indicators collected from individuals within communities. Discussion of the role of values in developing measures of quality of life is not stressed (although it is implied by the focus on community input) and the relationship of quality of life to social policy or social change is assumed.

THE DEVELOPMENTAL DISABILITIES APPROACH

The impetus for this work arose from a realization that many aspects of the lives of persons with disabilities were poor in quality. Among persons with developmental disabilities, the divergence between expectation and reality was so great as to require identification of broad areas of life functioning in need of attention.

Dimensions of Quality of Life in the Developmental Disabilities
Literature

Schalock's (1990b) quality of life taxonomy illustrates the breadth of
areas encompassed within a broadened quality of life framework. It
outlines six areas, namely self-esteem, social; self-esteem, beauty; self-
direction (independence); social relations; environmental comfort and
convenience; and safety and security. Each of these areas cuts across
three settings: home, community, and work or production. For example,
social relations at home involves family, social relations in the community involves friends, and at the workplace, co-workers. Similarly, safety
and security across the three settings involves food and shelter, safe
community, and a safe workplace and sufficient income.

The work in the developmental disabilities area is broad in both its
scope and implications. There is a greater awareness of the breadth
of quality of life issues, an emphasis on personal control, independence, and personal empowerment, as well as a greater willingness
to engage in discussions of the social policy implications of quality of
life assessments (Renwick et al., 1996). Many of these implications are
explicitly stated (e.g., Schalock, 1990b). In addition, there is a balanced
orientation towards objective and subjective indicators of quality of
life. There is a balanced emphasis upon individual and system-level
indicators and the importance of values in measurement is explicitly
emphasized. Quality of life measurement is assumed to be tied to
social policy and change goals.

THE SOCIAL INDICATORS APPROACH

Most quality of life approaches have a strong individual focus. For a
number of reasons, including interest in the determinants of health
(Evans et al., 1994), the impact of the *Healthy Cities* and *Healthy
Communities* movements (Ashton, 1992; Davies and Kelly, 1993), and
growing concern with consumers' views of health and social service
resources and provision, more attention is being directed to environmental indicators of quality of life. The social indicators literature
contains many suggestions for those who wish to focus upon quality
of life at a systems level.

Rationale for Social Indicators

During the 1960s interest in social indicators surged in both North America and Europe as a means of providing evidence on the impact of government social programs (Land, 1975). An initial definition of social indicators was presented in *Towards a Social Report* (U.S. Department of Health, Education, and Welfare, 1969):

> A social indicator, as the term is used here, may be defined to be a statistic of direct normative interest which facilitates concise, comprehensive and balanced judgments about the conditions of major aspects of a society. It is in all cases a direct measure of welfare and is subject to the interpretation that, if it changes in the "right" direction, while other things remain equal, things have gotten better, or people are "better off." Thus, statistics on the number of doctors or policemen could not be social indicators, whereas figures on health or crime rate could be. (p. 97)

Examples of Social Indicators with Quality of Life Implications

Early work (Sheldon and Land, 1972) suggested that the following could constitute the content categories of a social report using indicator systems: socioeconomic welfare, including population (composition, growth, and distribution); labor force and employment; income; knowledge and technology; education; health; leisure; public safety and legal system; housing; transportation; physical environment; social mobility and stratification. Social participation and alienation could also be assessed with focus upon: family; religion; politics; voluntary associations; and alienation. Finally, use of time, consumptive behaviour, aspiration, satisfaction, morale, and other characteristics of the population could be assessed.

The method of collecting these data could use objective measures of system functioning drawn from system-level data such as objective conditions (e.g., roles and social relations, income and consumption, and housing and safety). Individual-level measures in the form of subjective value-context measures (e.g., aspirations, expectations, and distributive justice value) or subjective well-being indices (e.g., life satisfaction, specific satisfaction, and alienation) could be employed.

Individual and societal level examples. One contemporary individual-level approach is that of the *Swedish Level of Living Surveys* (Erikson, 1993). Indicators used include: health and access to health care, employment and working conditions, economic resources, and education and skills.

Community-level indicators. An extensive literature has now accumulated that addresses the quality of life of communities. Many studies have reported residents' scores on researcher-designed instruments. These include North American studies of perceived neighbourhood quality (Connerly and Marans, 1985; Furuseth and Walcott, 1990; Olsen et al., 1985) as well as analyses based in Switzerland (Walter-Busch, 1983), South Africa (Moller and Schlemmer, 1983), Norway (Mastekaasa and Mourn, 1984), and Sweden (Tahlin, 1990).

In relation to the four quality of life measurement issues initially mentioned, the social indicators approach has a balanced orientation towards objective and subjective indicators of functioning. There is a balanced emphasis upon individual and system-level indicators with greater emphasis on system-level data. The importance of values in measurement is explicit and emphasized. Indicator measurement is assumed to be tied to social policy and goals for social change.

THE CENTRE FOR HEALTH PROMOTION MODEL

The next approach we consider is the model of quality of life developed by researchers at the Centre for Health Promotion, University of Toronto. The work builds upon a focus on health rather than illness, the WHO emphasis on health as a resource for daily living (WHO, 1986), and work in the developmental disabilities field.

Our conceptualization defines quality of life as: *The degree to which a person enjoys the important possibilities of his/her life.* Enjoyment encompasses two meanings: experience of subjective satisfaction and the possession or achievement of some characteristic or state, as, for example, in the phrase: "She enjoys a good standard of living." Possibilities reflect the opportunities and limitations each person has.

Quality of life is the degree of enjoyment that results from possibilities that have taken on importance to the person; that is, quality of life is uniquely identified for each individual.

There are three life domains: Being, Belonging, and Becoming. Being reflects "who one is" and has three subdomains: physical, psychological, and spiritual Being. Physical Being encompasses physical health, personal hygiene, nutrition, exercise, grooming, clothing, and general physical appearance. Psychological Being includes the person's psychological health and adjustment, cognitions, feelings, and evaluations concerning the self such as self-esteem, self-concept, and self-control. Spiritual Being refers to the personal values, personal standards of conduct, and spiritual beliefs that one holds.

The Belonging domain concerns the person's fit with his/her environments and also has three sub-domains. Physical Belonging describes the person's connections with his/her physical environments of home, workplace, neighbourhood, school, and community. Social Belonging includes links with social environments and involves acceptance by intimate others, family, friends, co-workers, and neighbourhood and community. Community Belonging represents access to resources such as adequate income, health and social services, employment, educational and recreational programs, and community events and activities.

Becoming refers to the purposeful activities carried out to express oneself and to achieve personal goals, hopes, and aspirations. Practical Becoming describes day-to-day activities such as domestic activities, paid work, school or volunteer activities, and seeing to health or social needs. Leisure Becoming includes activities that promote relaxation and stress reduction. Growth Becoming activities promote the maintenance or improvement of knowledge and skills and adapting to change.

In relation to the four quality of life measurement issues, there is a strong orientation towards subjective indicators of functioning at the individual level. Discussion concerning issues of the role of values in developing measures of quality of life is given much importance. To date, the examination of the implication of quality of life findings to social policy or social change is only in the development phase, but the potential for such impact is very strong (see Renwick and Brown, 1996).

LINDSTROM'S QUALITY OF LIFE MODEL

The final model we consider is one of the few psychologically oriented models that explicitly directs attention to system-level issues. More specifically, Lindstrom's model (1992, 1994) examines four spheres. The Personal sphere includes physical, mental, and spiritual resources, and the Interpersonal sphere includes family structure and function, intimate friends, and extended social networks. These are the areas usually considered in discussions of quality of life and health issues and Lindstrom examines these areas through large-scale surveys.

The External sphere includes aspects of work, income, and housing. The Global sphere includes the societal macro environment, specific cultural aspects, and human rights and social welfare policies. It is in this latter area, with its analysis, usually through policy analysis, of distribution of societal resources and general social welfare approaches, where some of the most interesting determinants of health may be uncovered. Lindstrom analyzes Nordic children's health in relation to these latter spheres. Readers are urged to obtain his monograph. These kinds of policy analysis are infrequently carried out within a quality of life framework and offer potential areas of multidisciplinary integration.

IMPLICATIONS FOR THE QUALITY OF LIFE AND HEALTH AGENDA

The Centre for Health Promotion's quality of life model directs attention to a broad range of issues including personal development opportunities, immediate environments, and community resources. The model has served as a heuristic for identifying issues related to the health of seniors (Raphael et al., 1995) and adolescents (Raphael, 1996a; Raphael, 1996b), and general health promotion and rehabilitation issues (Renwick et al., 1996). The strong multidisciplinary conceptual framework helps identify areas of further inquiry.

Lindstrom's model highlights the importance of considering societal and structural determinants of health. Most researchers in the quality of life and health area work within an individual perspective and tend to ignore broader social determinants of health. Lindstrom has been one of the few to consider broader issues as they pertain to health issues. Analysis of the social determinants of health, including broader societal factors, is now an active area of inquiry in health promotion and related disciplines.

UPDATE: CURRENT STATUS AND EMERGING CONCEPTIONS

There have been some interesting developments in the quality of life indicators and health area since 1996. The most obvious has been the continuing emphasis upon health-related quality of life in the academic literature. Any search in Google Scholar, for example, using the term "quality of life" brings up a multitude of focused research articles on patient responses to numerous diseases and the quality of life effects on patients of various forms of treatment.

The applications of the quality of life model developed by the Centre for Health Promotion continued to be developed and much of the material that follows details these activities. To our knowledge, no model that matches this approach in complexity and detail has been developed since the original publication of this paper. The Quality of Life Research Unit at the University of Toronto continues to make available the various scales and carries on with research applications of the model.

The social indicators field, however, has seen an important expansion in the development and application of international comparative policy-related indicators. Particularly noteworthy have been the Report Cards on Children's Health by UNICEF's Innocenti Research Centre in Florence and the reports of the Organisation for Economic Co-operation and Development (OECD). Especially useful has been the OECD *Society at a Glance, Health at a Glance,* and *Education at a Glance* series, among others. The United Nations Human Development Program's annual report cards also provide a wealth of indicator data that can be used to inform public policymaking. Details concerning these developments are contained in the materials in this volume. See especially the recommended readings and websites.

REFERENCES

Ashton, J.: 1992, Healthy Cities (Open University Press, Philadelphia).

Bowling, A.: 1991, Measuring Health: A review of quality of life instruments (Open University Press, Philadelphia).

Brown, R. I., M. B. Bayer, and P. M. Brown: 1992, Empowerment and Developmental Handicaps: Choices and Quality of Life (Captus Press, Toronto).

Connerly, C. E. and R. W. Marans: 1985, 'Comparing two global measures of perceived neighbourhood quality'. Social Indicators Research 17, pp. 29–47.

Davies, J. K. and M. P. Kelly: 1993, Healthy Cities: Research and Practice (Routledge, New York).

Erikson, R.: 1993, 'Descriptions of inequality: The Swedish approach to welfare research', in M. Nussbaum and A. Sen (eds.), The Quality of Life (Clarendon Press, Oxford).

Evans, R. G., M. Barer and T. R. Marmor: 1994, Why Are Some People Healthy and Others Not? The Determinants of Health of Populations (Aldine de Gruyter, New York).

Furuseth, O. and W. A. Walcott: 1990, 'Defining quality of life in North Carolina', The Social Science Journal 27, pp. 75–93.

Goode, D.: 1994, Quality of Life for Persons with Disabilities: International Issues and Perspectives (Brookline Press, Cambridge, MA).

Green, L. and M. Kreuter: 1991, Health Promotion Planning (Mayfield, Toronto).

Hollandsworth, J.: 1988, 'Evaluating the impact of medical treatment on the quality of life: A 5 year update', Social Science and Medicine 26, pp. 425–434.

Land, K. C.: 1975, 'Social indicator models: An overview', in K. C. Land and S. Spilerman (eds.), Social Indicator Models (Russell Sage Foundation, New York).

Lindstrom, B.: 1992, Quality of life: A model for evaluating "Health for All." Soz Praventivmed 37, pp. 301–306.

Lindstrom, B.: 1994, The Essence of Existence: On the Quality of Life of Children in the Nordic Countries (The Nordic School of Public Health, Goteborg, Sweden).

Livneh, H.: 1988, 'Rehabilitation goals: their hierarchical and multifaceted nature', Journal of Applied Rehabilitation Counselling 19(3), pp. 12–18.

Mastekaasa, A. and T. Mourn: 1984, 'The perceived quality of life in Norway: Regional variations and contextual effects', Social Indicators Research 14, pp. 385–419.

McDowell, I. and C. Newell: 1987, Measuring Health (Oxford University Press, New York).

Moller, V. and L. Schlemmer: 1983, 'Quality of life in South Africa: Towards an instrument for the assessment of quality of life and basic needs', Social Indicators Research 12, pp. 225–279.

Naess, S.: 1987, Quality of Life Research: Concepts, Methods, and Applications (Institute of Applied Social Research, Oslo, Norway).

Olsen, M. E., P. Canan and M. Hennessy: 1985, 'A value-based community assessment process: Integrating quality of life and social impact studies', Sociological Methods and Research 13, pp. 325–361.

Parmenter, T.: 1994, 'Quality of life as a concept and measurable entity', Social Indicators Research 33, pp. 9–46.

Raphael, D.: 1996a, 'Determinants of health of North American adolescents: Evolving definitions, recent findings, and proposed research agenda', Journal of Adolescent Health 19, pp. 6–16.

Raphael, D.: 1996b, 'Quality of life and adolescent health', in R. Renwick, I. Brown and M. Nagler (eds.), Quality of Life in Health Promotion and Rehabilitation: Conceptual Approaches, Issues, and Applications (Sage Publications, Thousand Oaks, CA).

Raphael, D., I. Brown, R. Renwick, M. Cava, K. Heathcote, and N. Weir: 1995, 'The quality of life of seniors living in the community: A conceptualization with implications for public health practice', Canadian Journal of Public Health 86, pp. 228–233.

Raphael, D., I. Brown, R. Renwick, and I. Rootman: 1994, Quality of Life Theory and Assessment: What are the Implications for Health Promotion? Issues in Health Promotion Monograph Series (Centre for Health Promotion, University of Toronto and ParticipACTION, Toronto).

Renwick, R. and I. Brown: 1996, 'Being, belonging, becoming: the Centre for Health Promotion model of quality of life', in R. Renwick, I. Brown, and M. Nagler (eds.), Quality of Life in Health Promotion and Rehabilitation: Conceptual Approaches, Issues, and Applications (Sage Publications, Thousand Oaks, CA).

Renwick, R., I. Brown, and M. Nagler (eds.): 1996, Quality of Life in Health Promotion and Rehabilitation: Conceptual Approaches, Issues, and Applications (Sage Publications, Thousand Oaks, CA).

Romney, E., R. Brown, R., and P. Fry (eds.): 1994, 'Improving the quality of life of people with and without disabilities', [Special Issue]. Social Indicators Research 33 (1–3).

Schalock, R. L.: 1990a, Quality of life: Perspective and Issues (American Association on Mental Retardation, Washington, DC).

Schalock, R. L.: 1990b, 'Where do we go from here?', in R. Schalock (ed.), Quality of Life: Perspective and Issues (American Association on Mental Retardation, Washington, DC).

Schipper, H., J. Clinch, and V. Powell: 1990, 'Definitions and conceptual issues', in B. Spilker (ed.), Quality of Life in Clinical Trials (Raven, New York).

Sheldon, E. and K. C. Land: 1972, 'Social reporting for the 1970's: A review and programmatic statement', Policy Sciences 3, pp. 137–151.

Spilker, B.: 1990, Quality of Life in Clinical Trials (Raven, New York).

Stewart, A. and J. Ware: 1992, Measuring Functioning and Well-Being: The Medical Outcome Study Approach (Duke University Press, Durham NC).

Tahlin, M.: 1990, 'Politics, dynamics, and individualism—The Swedish approach to level of living research', Social Indicators Research 22, pp. 155–180.

Thorndike, E. L: 1939, Your City (Harcourt, Brace and Company, New York).

U.S. Department of Health, Education, and Welfare: 1969, Towards a Social Report (U.S. Governmental Printing Office, Washington, DC).

Walter-Busch, E.: 1983, 'Subjective and objective indicators of regional quality of life in Switzerland', Social Indicators Research 12, pp. 337–391.

World Health Organization: 1986, Ottawa Charter on Health Promotion (WHO, Geneva, Switzerland).

CHAPTER 3

Quality of Life: What are the Implications for Health Promotion?

Dennis Raphael, Ivan Brown, Rebecca Renwick, and Irving Rootman

Quality of life (QOL) is concerned with what makes for the "good life." Philosophers have long been interested in this question, but empirical research in QOL had, until quite recently, been the focus primarily of sociologists, social psychologists, and economists.[1,2] There is disagreement on how it should be defined, and this disagreement occurs within all fields where it has been used.[3] QOL has been applied to wellness and health,[4] the impact of illness,[5] availability of financial resources,[6] work life and leisure,[7-10] life roles,[11] culture,[12] community concerns,[13] and community integration.[14] There has also been disagreement on whether QOL is primarily an objective or a subjective phenomenon.[15]

Table 3.1 provides a summary of recent QOL conceptualizations.

As health promoters concerned with broader determinants of health, we felt that available conceptualizations of QOL were not particularly useful for health promoters. More specifically, these approaches focused unduly on illness and disability, defined QOL domains much too narrowly, and assumed that the basic dimensions of QOL differed between age groups; that is, one model existed for seniors, another for adolescents, another for persons with developmental disabilities, and so forth. Our conceptualization was guided by the principles that the components of QOL are the same for *all* people; QOL should be broadly conceived and include physical, psychological, spiritual, social, and environmental dimensions; and control and opportunities are important components of QOL.

THE CENTRE FOR HEALTH PROMOTION (CHP) MODEL

We were initially asked by the Ontario (Canada) Ministry of Community and Social Services to develop a conceptual model and instrumentation for assessing the QOL of persons with developmental disabilities. This framework would be used to evaluate the Ministry's long-term plan for promoting community-based living and services for those with these disabilities.[16] This project was not initially conceived as a health promotion study, yet within the broadened World Health Organization definition of health,[17] our QOL approach was clearly working within a health promotion perspective.

Table 3.1: Various Definitions of Quality of Life

Approach	Focus	Definition
Medical	Persons with diseases	Quality of life represents the functional effect of an illness and its consequent therapy upon a patient, as perceived by the patient.[5]
Health related	Persons with illness or disabilities	Quality of life is recognized as a concept representing individual responses to the physical, mental, and social effects of illness on daily living that influence the extent to which personal satisfaction with life circumstances can be achieved.[4]
Social diagnosis	Persons in communities	... the adjustment and life satisfaction of community members.[13]
Developmental disabilities	Persons with developmental disabilities	Quality of life is the outcome of individuals meeting basic needs and fulfilling basic responsibilities in community settings (family, recreational, school, and work).[14]
Aging	Persons aged 55+	Quality of life is the multidimensional evaluation, by both intrapersonal and social-normative criteria, of the person-environment system of an individual in time past, current, and anticipated.[15]
Social indicators	Societies or communities	Statistics of direct normative interest that facilitates concise, comprehensive, and balanced judgments about the conditions of major aspects of society.[6]

Defining QOL

The CHP conceptual approach was broadly influenced by the humanistic-existential tradition.[18-22] A detailed discussion of these philosophical foundations appears elsewhere,[23] but, by way of summary, this literature recognizes that individuals have physical, psychological, and spiritual dimensions.[19] It also acknowledges people's need to belong, in a physical and a social sense (i.e., to places and social groups),[18] as well as to distinguish themselves as individuals by pursuing their own goals and making their own choices and decisions.[18,24] QOL is defined as "The degree to which a person enjoys the important possibilities of his/her life." The enjoyment of important possibilities is relevant to three major life domains: *Being*, *Belonging*, and *Becoming*. These are described below.

The Being, Belonging, and Becoming Content Domains

Being reflects "who one is" and has three subdomains. *Physical Being* encompasses physical health, personal hygiene, nutrition, exercise, grooming, clothing, and general appearance. *Psychological Being* includes the person's psychological health and adjustment, cognitions, feelings, and evaluations concerning the self, such as self-esteem and self-concept. *Spiritual Being* refers to one's personal values, standards of conduct, and spiritual beliefs.

The *Belonging* domain concerns the person's fit with his or her environments and also has three subdomains. *Physical Belonging* describes the person's connections with the physical environments of home, workplace, neighbourhood, school, and community. *Social Belonging* includes links with social environments and involves acceptance by intimate others, family, friends, co-workers, and neighborhood and community. *Community Belonging* represents access to public resources, such as adequate income, health and social services, employment, educational and recreational programs, and community events and activities.

Becoming refers to the activities carried out in the course of daily living, including those to achieve personal goals, hopes, and aspirations. *Practical Becoming* describes day-to-day activities, such as domestic activities, paid work, school, or volunteer activities, and seeing to health or social needs. *Leisure Becoming* includes activities carried out primarily for enjoyment that promote relaxation and stress reduction. *Growth Becoming* activities promote the maintenance or improvement of knowledge and skills, and adapting to change.

Enjoyment of possibilities has two aspects: experiencing satisfaction or pleasure and possession or attainment of something, as in the statement "She enjoys a comfortable standard of living." These two aspects of enjoyment are closely related. The extent of a person's QOL in the domains is determined by two factors: importance and enjoyment. Thus, QOL consists of the relative importance or meaning attached to each particular dimension and the extent of the person's enjoyment.

WHY IS THE QOL MODEL RELEVANT TO HEALTH PROMOTION?

We believe that there are four, somewhat overlapping reasons why our approach is relevant for health promotion. The domains of QOL may serve as a determinant of health; improvement in the domains may be seen as a desired goal of health promotion activities; assessment within the domains can serve as an indicator of needs; and our model draws attention to the role of environments in supporting the promotion of health.

QOL as a Determinant of Health

One way of looking at QOL is to consider it as a determinant of health. The central idea here is that better QOL leads to improved health and that poor QOL results in reduced physical, mental, and social well-being. In the seniors area, for example, Raphael[25] and Raphael, Brown, Renwick, Cava, Weir, et al.[26] summarize evidence that significant differences in functioning occur among seniors even in the absence of medical pathology. These differences have been described as involving the distinction between pathological, normative, and optimal aging.[27-29]

Normal aging is the typical process in any given society; optimal aging occurs under development-enhancing and age-friendly environmental conditions; and sick or pathological aging is characterized by medical etiology and illness. Support for this distinction comes from demographic studies of lifestyle and health relationships,[30,31] social support and health,[32,33] and studies of cognitive functioning across the age span.[34] These extra-individual factors are often categorized as "quality of life" components.[13,35,36]

It appears that seniors' functioning associated with normal aging in Western countries is well below achievable levels. Further, it is clear that many determinants of health show overlap with the QOL dimensions and domains found in the literature. Similarly, it is difficult to avoid the conclusion that QOL informs the literature on health status among other populations. QOL provides a context for understanding specific adolescent behaviors, such as smoking and drinking behavior, sexual behavior, and delinquency,[37] as well as general coping.[38]

A recent analysis considered the determinants of adolescent health within the CHP QOL framework.[39] The health gradients related to socioeconomic status,[40-42] and the persistence of health problems among Aboriginal, poor, and other marginalized populations provides other examples of this relationship.[43]

QOL as an Outcome of Health Promotion Interventions

The definition of health as a resource for living suggests that improved QOL is an outcome of health maintenance and health promotion activities. Further, it appears that many of the goals and objectives of health promotion programs involve QOL issues as we define them. For example, the mandatory programs for Healthy Elderly put out by the Ontario (Canada) Ministry of Health[44] call for health departments to focus on health promotion and disease prevention; enhance coping; promote self-care; facilitate empowerment and promote independence; create positive social environments; and plan healthy physical environments. For Green and Kreuter, QOL is the beginning and end point of health education and promotion interventions.[13]

QOL as an Indicator of Need

A QOL focus causes policy makers, health promoters, and consumers to reflect upon the essence of everyday life. This may sound somewhat metaphysical, but we seldom take time to consider what really is important in individuals' lives and reflect on a society's responsibilities to provide a "quality life" for all of its citizens. A focus upon QOL issues directs attention to needed social policy and service provision reform.[45] This argument suggests potential usefulness in a range of needs analysis activities.

QOL and the Role of Environments

Our QOL model directs attention to environments. Many aspects of life quality are concerned with environmental and societal factors in addition to personal characteristics, such as attitudes, beliefs, and personal behaviors. QOL reflects individuals' perceptions of and responses to environments, thereby directing attention to the impact of the policies and services of governments and other institutions upon individuals' QOL.[46]

APPLICATIONS OF THE MODEL

These concepts have been operationalized for various population groups. Instrumentation has been developed and validated for persons with developmental disabilities,[18] seniors living in the community,[29] and adolescents.[48] The development of each instrument included an examination of the relevance of the domains for each population, significant input from the population of interest in creating items, and an ongoing validation process.[48]

PERSONS WITH DEVELOPMENTAL DISABILITIES

The assessment of QOL of persons with developmental disabilities is a complex task. It is especially important because a great many aspects of their lives are affected by service policy or programming changes.[49] Our measurement approach calls for a multimethod, multisource approach. At least half a day is spent with the person with disabilities and at least an hour with a significant other person, either a service provider or parent. The assessor also provides an overall QOL assessment. Three measures collect information from the person with disabilities.

Participant Interview

This measure is a semistructured interview that provides a flexible format for gathering the person's perceptions. Each of the nine sub-domains is broken down into six concepts. The assessor asks 54 key questions—six for each of the nine areas of life—and may ask a number of follow-up probes. *Importance* and *Enjoyment* are rated by the assessor on a 5-point scale. The QOL of each participant comes from the unique pattern of responses to the 54 key questions. To illustrate, for Physical Being the six concepts are physical health, eating a balanced diet, physical mobility, hygiene and body care, personal appearance, and activity level and fitness. The key questions for these concepts are:

1) Tell me about your health, how you feel.
2) What food do you usually eat?
3) Tell me about getting around. Can you move around like you want to?
4) What do you do to be neat and clean?
5) What do you like about the way you look? and
6) What exercise do you get?

The probes for the first key question physical health, are:

1) Are you ever sick?
2) When do you feel the best?
3) Do you have a doctor? A dentist?
4) When do you go?
5) What do you do to be more healthy?
6) Is looking after your health important to you?
7) How important? and
8) Are you happy with how healthy you are?

Self-ratings

The people with developmental disabilities provide their own perceptions of their QOL. Sets of four items (one set for each of the nine subdomains of QOL) inquire into the Importance, Enjoyment, Control, and Opportunities for a domain. Responses for Importance and Enjoyment are along a 5-point scale, whereas the Control and Opportunities components are assessed using three categories. To illustrate, for the subdomain of Physical Being the person with developmental disabilities responds to:

1) Do you care what you look like? (Importance)

2) Do you like the way you look? (Enjoyment)

3) Who decides what clothes you wear? (Control) and

4) If you wanted to, could you look different? (Opportunities)

Personal Control Questionnaire

Participants are asked whether they can influence decisions concerning their lives in six areas: where they live; daily activities; how they use their spending money; how they enjoy themselves; what foods they eat; and what time they go to bed. For each area, one question asks who makes or made the decision, and another inquires into whether changes in this situation are possible.

Data from a Close Other

OTHER-PERSON QUESTIONNAIRE

Each of the nine areas of QOL is broken down into six concepts—the same concepts contained in the *Participant Interview*. For each concept, ratings for Importance, Enjoyment, Control, and Opportunities are provided, through a paper-and-pencil format by the close-other person, regarding their perceptions of the life of the person with developmental disabilities.

PERSONAL-CONTROL QUESTIONNAIRE

This is the same instrument administered to the person with developmental disabilities.

Data from the Assessor

The assessor completes an *Assessor Checklist* based on minimal standards for commonly held expectations for individuals' QOL, such as cleanliness, hygiene, diet, social contacts, and problem solving. Assessors draw upon their observations, results of the interview, and informal conversations with significant people in the lives of the persons with developmental disabilities to make these ratings.

A *QOL Profile* is developed for each individual. Collecting QOL data from persons with developmental disabilities is the main focus, but data from other persons provide important contextual information within which to interpret data from the person with disabilities. Perceptions of a person's QOL may differ between sources, and these differences are not seen as reflecting measurement error as much as divergence in valid perceptions between individuals. When divergence occurs, inquiry is undertaken to analyze the source of these differences.

Reliability/Validity and Pilot-implementation Study

The Ministry of Community and Social Services provided funding for a reliability/validity and pilot-implementation study. A study of 90 subjects found the instruments to be reliable and valid.[16] A range of analyses assessed the internal consistencies (Cronbach alpha) of the domains, degree of agreement between interviewers, and test-retest of client responses (most coefficients >.90). Instrument scores were correlated with each other as well as with an external criterion measure, the Schalock Quality of Life Scale.[14] An extensive survey of 500+ persons with developmental disabilities in the province of Ontario is now underway.

SENIORS LIVING IN THE COMMUNITY

The Health Promotion for Seniors Working Group of the North York Community Health Promotion Research Unit reviewed and accepted the CHP model of QOL as a basis for using it for assessing QOL of seniors in the community. We focused upon community-living seniors who could provide self-report concerning QOL. The Seniors and an additional Adolescents applications are presented in Chapters 4 and 5.

COMMUNITY-LEVEL INDICATORS OF QOL

We have been asking Toronto residents: *What is it about your community or neighbourhood that makes life better for you and the people you care about?* These data are being used to develop community-level models of QOL. This work is presented as Chapters 6 and 7.

HOW CAN QOL CONSIDERATIONS INFORM HEALTH PROMOTION PRACTICE?

In this section, we explore how our model could be applied by health promoters. Three general approaches to health promotion activities are usually outlined: social policy, community based, and individual based.[50] Although the pendulum of popularity swings back and forth among these approaches, it seems clear that each has a role in promoting health and improving QOL.

Social Policy Approaches

These approaches to health promotion are defined as "ecological in perspective, multi-sectorial in scope and participatory in strategy."[51] We have identified QOL areas with obvious social policy implications. Among seniors, for example, dental care becomes more important at a time of life when many are least able to afford it. Poor dental care has consequences for nutrition, appearance, social interaction, and general life satisfaction. These issues are relevant as well for adolescents whose families may not be able to afford quality care. Social policy questions include:

1) Should free dental care be available to seniors or others with low incomes?

2) Could special discounts be provided to support dental health?

Another example of an important issue for seniors and persons with disabilities is access to public transit and adequate housing. How can accessibility be increased? Would improved access improve other QOL areas?

Community-based Approaches

Community-mobilization approaches target and organize members of a common geographical, social, or cultural unit for health-promotion activities. Community development approaches place a greater emphasis upon strengthening communities through community members' identification and solution of self-defined problems.[52] The connectedness of individuals with their environments is an important focus of both of these community-level approaches. Connectedness with environments is an important part of our QOL model. Individuals' lack of sense of physical, social, and community belonging can indicate need; improved belonging resulting from activities can be an indicator of program success.

Additionally, many aspects of day-to-day, leisure, and growth or maintenance activities, especially among seniors and adolescents, are not only identified as important issues, but frequently are also the focus of community-level interventions. These practical, leisure, and growth issues are also highlighted by a QOL approach and may best be influenced through community-based activities.

Individual-level Approaches

Many health service and health promoters continue to work individually with consumers. People are treated for illness or disability, public health departments identify individuals at risk, and physicians continue to see clients one at a time. Such one-on-one opportunities can be used to inquire into QOL. Individuals can be provided with information and knowledge that can enhance QOL. A QOL focus includes both identifying a range of issues that impact a person's life and working with the person on these issues to improve one's QOL.

CONCLUSIONS

QOL may be a determinant of health among populations and may well help differentiate between healthy and nonhealthy functioning individuals. QOL should serve as an important outcome of health promotion activities. Because QOL can be improved through social policy, community-based, or individual-level activities, a QOL approach provides a useful way to conceptualize domains of functioning and identify targets of health-promoting activities.

A variety of applications can draw upon our model. Within the disabilities area, the model can be used directly with individuals and groups (i.e., those sharing a residence or workshop). QOL assessments can identify areas in which persons are experiencing good or poor QOL and can inform program planning and intervention. Assessments can then evaluate the efficacy of these interventions. Renwick, Brown, and Raphael[53] provide further service implications of a QOL focus.

With seniors and adolescents, QOL assessments can determine health, health promotion, and service needs. Our work with seniors and adolescents has identified areas of need that can be addressed by local public health departments. To date, seniors and adolescents have completed paper-and-pencil instruments, but the profiles could be administered through face-to-face administration or telephone surveys.

Short (54 items) and brief (27 items) versions of the Seniors Profile have been developed and validated[54] for research and screening purposes. Raphael and McClelland outline a range of QOL applications for health promotion activities with seniors.[55] Raphael et al. have done the same for adolescents.[47] Finally, local communities are considering use of the community-level model for assessing community needs in order to plan health promotion programs and activities.[56]

UPDATE

The time since the original publication of this article has seen the QOL model refined and extended to inquiry at a variety of levels. Following the creation of numerous QOL measures designed to assess QOL among persons with disabilities, adolescents, and seniors, a community QOL approach was developed and applied. The approach was then extended to consider how public policymaking was influencing QOL. These developments are documented in the following sections of this volume.

The health promotion field has continued to develop and numerous key volumes and articles have appeared. Particularly noteworthy are the second edition of *Health Promotion in Canada*[57] and a special issue of *Critical Public Health* that reviews developments since the Ottawa Charter.[58] However, there is increasing concern about whether health promotion remains a significant influence upon health-related activity in Canada.[58]

Governmental unwillingness to address the prerequisites of health combined with a continuing societal focus on individually oriented risk factors such as tobacco and alcohol use, physical inactivity, and poor nutrition related to lack of ingestion of fruits and vegetables have left little space for a broad approach to health as advanced by health promotion. The rise of the "obesity epidemic" also distracts from the concerns of health promotion. Much of the material in this volume concerns itself with how health promotion can contribute to improving the QOL of Canadians in light of these developments.

REFERENCES

1. Lindstrom, B. Quality of life: A model for evaluating "Health for All." Conceptual considerations and policy implications. *Sozial- und Präventivmedizin* 1992;37:301–306.

2. Woodill, G. Renwick, R. Brown, I. Raphael, D. Being, belonging and becoming: An approach to the quality of life of persons with development disabilities. In Goode, D. ed. *Quality of Life for Persons with Disabilities: International Issues and Perspectives*. Boston, MA: Brookline Press, 1994.

3. Raphael, D. Quality of life: Eleven debates concerning its measurement. In Renwick, R. Brown. I., Nagler, N., eds. *Quality of Life in Health Promotion and Rehabilitation: Conceptual Approaches, Issues, and Applications*. Thousand Oaks, CA: Sage, 1996.

4. Bowling, A. *Measuring Health*. Philadelphia, PA: Open University Press, 1991.

5. Schipper, H., Clinch, J., Powell, V. Definitions and conceptual issues. In Spilker, B., ed. *Quality of Life in Clinical Trials*. New York: Raven, 1990.

6. Andrews, F.M. Introduction. In Andrews, F.M. ed. *Research on the Quality of Life*. Ann Arbor, MI: Institute for Social Research, 1986.

7. Brief, A., Hollenback, J. Work and the quality of life. *International Journal of Psychology* 1985;20:199–206.

8. Czikszentmihalyi, M., LeFevre, J. Optimal experience in work and leisure. *Journal of Personality and Social Psychology* 1989;56:815–822.

9. Near, J., Rice, R., Hunt, R. Job satisfaction and life satisfaction: A profile analysis. *Social Indicators Research* 1987;19:383–401.

10. Shamir, B., Saloman, I., Work-at-home and quality of working life. *Academy of Management Review* 1985;10:455–464.

11. McLanahan, F., Adams, S. Parenthood and psychological well-being. *Annual Review of Sociology* 1987;13:237–257.

12. Hayashi, C., Suzuki, T., Hayashi, F. Comparative study of lifestyles and quality of life: Japan and France. *Behavioumetrika* 1984;15:1–17.

13. Green, L., Kreuter, M., *Health Promotion Planning.* Toronto, ON: Mayfield, 1991.

14. Schalock, R. ed. *Quality of Life: Perspectives and Issues.* Washington, DC: American Association on Mental Retardation, 1990.

15. Lawton, M.P. A multidimensional view of quality of life in frail elders. In Birren. J., Lubben, I., Rowe, J., Deutchman D., eds, *The Concept and Measurement of Quality of Life in the Frail Elderly.* New York: Academic Press, 1991.

16. Raphael, D., Brown, I., Renwick, R., Rootman, I. Assessing the quality of life of persons with developmental disabilities: Description of a new model, measuring instruments, and initial findings. *International Journal of Disability, Development, and Education* 1996;43:25–42.

17. World Health Organization. *Constitution.* Geneva: WHO, 1946.

18. Bakan, D. *The Duality of Human Existence: Isolation and Communion in Western Man.* Boston, MA: Beacon, 1964.

19. Becker E. *The Birth and Death of Meaning,* 2nd ed. New York: Free Press, 1971.

20. Merleau-Ponty, J. *The Visible and the Invisible.* Evanston, IL: Northwestern University Press, 1968.

21. Sullivan, E. *A Critical Psychology: Interpretation of the Personal World.* New York: Plenum, 1984.

22. Zaner, R. *The Context of Self: A Phenomenological Inquiry Using Medicine as a Clue.* Athens, OH: Ohio University Press, 1981.

23. Renwick, R., Brown, I. Being, belonging, becoming: The Centre for Health Promotion model of quality of life. In Renwick, R. Brown, I., Nagler, M., eds., *Quality of Life in Health Promotion and Rehabilitation: Conceptual Approaches, Issues, and Applications.* Thousand Oaks, CA: Sage, 1996.

24. Bourdieu, P. *Outline of a Theory of Practice.* London: Cambridge University Press, 1977.

25. Raphael, D. Quality of life of older adults: Towards the optimization of the aging process. In Renwick, R., Brown, I., Nagler, N. eds., *Quality of Life in Health Promotion and Rehabilitation: Conceptual Approaches, Issues, and Applications.* Thousand Oaks, CA: Sage, 1996.

26. Raphael, D., Brown, I., Renwick, R., Cava, M. Weir, N., et al. The quality of life of seniors living in the community: A conceptualization with implications for public health practice. *Canadian Journal of Public Health* 1995;86:228-233.

27. Baltes, P., Baltes, M. Psychological perspectives on successful aging: The model of selective optimization with compensation. In Baltes, P., Baltes, M., eds., *Successful Aging: Perspectives from the Social Sciences.* New York: Cambridge University Press, 1990.

28. Rowe, J., Kahn, R. Human aging: Usual and successful. *Science* 1987;237: 143-149.

29. Whitbourne, S.K. *The Aging Body.* New York: Springer, 1985.

30. Berkman, L.F., Breslow, L. *Health and Ways of Living: The Alameda County Study.* New York: Oxford University Press, 1983.

31. Kaplan, G., Haan, M.P. Is there a role for prevention among the elderly: Epidemiological evidence from the Alameda county study. In Ory, M., Bond, K., eds. *Aging and Health Care: Social Science and Policy Perspectives.* New York: Routledge, 1989.

32. Berkman, L.F., Smye, SL. Social networks, host resistance, and mortality: A nine-year follow-up study of Alameda County residents. *American Journal of Epidemiology* 1979;109:186-204.

33. Cohen, S., Smye, S.L. *Social Support and Health.* Orlando, FL: Academic Press, 1985.

34. Schaie, K.W. The optimization of cognitive functioning in old age: Predications based on cohort-sequential and longitudinal data. In Baltes, P., Baltes, M., eds., *Successful Aging: Perspectives from The Social Sciences.* New York: Cambridge University Press, 1990.

35. Raphael, D., Brown, I., Renwick, R., Rootman, I. Quality of life theory and assessment: What are the implications for health promotion? *Issues in Health Promotion Monograph Series.* Toronto, ON: Centre for Health Promotion, University of Toronto and ParticipACTION, 1994.

36. Lindstrom, B. *The Essence of Existence: On the Quality of Life of Children in the Nordic Countries.* Goteborg, Sweden: The Nordic School of Public Health, 1994.

37. Office of Technology Assessment, U.S. Congress. *Adolescent Health.* Washington, DC: U.S. Congress, 1991.

38. Hurrelmann, K., Losel, F. *Health Hazards in Adolescence.* New York: de Gruyter, 1990.

39. Raphael, D. The determinants of adolescent health: Evolving definitions, recent findings, and proposed research agenda. *The Journal of Adolescent Health* 1996;19:6-16.

40. D'Arcy, C. Reducing inequalities in health: A review of literature. In *Knowledge Development for Health Promotion.* Ottawa, ON: Health and Welfare Canada, 1989.

41. McIntyre, S. The patterning of health by social position in contemporary Britain: Directions for sociological research. *Social Science and Medicine* 1986;23:393–415.

42. Rootman, I. Inequities in health: Sources and solutions. *Health Promotion* 1988;26(3):2–8.

43. Shan, C.P. *Public Health and Preventive Medicine in Canada*, 3rd edition. Toronto, ON: University of Toronto Press, 1994.

44. Ontario Ministry of Health. *Healthy Elderly: Principles and Program Strategies.* Toronto, ON: Public Health Branch, Ministry of Health, 1991.

45. Goode, D. ed. *Quality of Life for Persons with Disabilities: International Issues and Perspectives*. Boston, MA: Brookline Press, 1994.

46. Raphael, D. Quality of life and adolescent health. In Renwick, R., Brown, I., Nagler, N., eds. *Quality of Life in Health Promotion and Rehabilitation: Conceptual Approaches, Issues, and Applications*. Thousand Oaks, CA: Sage, 1996.

47. Raphael, D. Rukholm, E. Brown, I. Hill-Bailey, P. Donato, E. The quality of life profile—adolescent version: Background, description, and initial validation. *The Journal of Adolescent Health* 1996; 19:366–375.

48. Kassam, K. *Validating and Extending the Quality of Life Model in Group Health Activities with Non-English Speaking Seniors*. North York, ON: North York Community Health Promotion Research Unit Report Series, #96-02, 1996.

49. Raphael, D. Renwick, R. Brown, I. Studying the lives of persons with developmental disabilities: Methodological lessons from the quality of life project. *Journal on Developmental Disabilities* 1993;2(2):30–49.

50. Macdonald, G., Bunton, R. Health promotion: Discipline or disciplines? In Bunton, R., Macdonald, G., eds., *Health Promotion: Disciplines and Diversity*. London, UK: Routledge, 1992.

51. Milio, N. Making healthy public policy; developing the science by learning the art: An ecological framework for policy studies. *Health Promotion International* 1988;2:263–274.

52. Bracht, N. Introduction. In Bracht, N., ed. *Health Promotion at the Community Level*. Newbury Park, CA: Sage, 1990.

53. Renwick, R., Brown, I., Raphael, D. Quality of life: Linking a conceptual approach to service provision. *Journal on Developmental Disabilities* 1994;3(2):34–46.

54. Raphael, D., Smith, T., Brown, I., Renwick, R. Development and properties of the short and brief versions of the quality of life profile: Seniors version. *International Journal of Health Sciences* 1995;6:161–168.

55. Raphael, D., McClelland, B. Assessing the health and service needs of seniors, the quality of life profile, seniors version. *Public Health and Epidemiology Report, Ontario* 1994;6(5):125–127.

56. Raphael, D., Renwick, R., Rootman, I., Cho, S., Klimko, N, et al. *Development and Application of Community-Level Quality of life Indicators: A Community-Based Health Promotion Approach.* Toronto, ON: Centre For Health Promotion, 1996.

57. O'Neill, M., Pederson, A., Dupéré, S., Rootman, I., eds. *Health Promotion in Canada: Critical Perspectives.* Toronto, ON: Canadian Scholars' Press Inc., 2007.

58. Raphael, D. Grasping at straws: A recent history of health promotion in Canada. *Critical Public Health* 2008;18(4):483–495.

CHAPTER 4

The Quality of Life Profile—
Adolescent Version

Dennis Raphael, Ellen Rukholm, Ivan Brown, Pat Hill-Bailey, and Emily Donato

Adolescent health is becoming an important focus for North American health officials and researchers [1–4]. Mortality and morbidity rates for adolescents and young adults in Western countries have been increasing during the past few decades [5] and concern is especially great in the United States. There, attention has focused on the extent of adolescent involvement in unsettling behaviors, such as alcohol, tobacco, and other drug use, premature and unprotected sexual activity, and being either victims or perpetrators of violence [6]. In Canada, interest in adolescent health is related to the maturing of health-promotion perspectives [7,8] and the importance ascribed to developing stable health-promoting attitudes and habits prior to adulthood [9].

EXPANDED DEFINITIONS OF ADOLESCENT HEALTH

At a minimum, adolescent health now encompasses healthy behaviors in addition to health status [10,11]. Healthy behaviors reduce immediate risk and support the development of stable health-related lifestyles. There is also increased willingness to consider aspects of adolescent coping and adolescent development within these formulations [12]. The concept of quality of life could provide a framework within which aspects of adolescent health could be examined [13,14].

A quality of life perspective is useful for several reasons [15]. Since quality of life approaches usually integrate psychologic and sociologic perspectives, issues usually neglected by health workers trained within the medical, nursing, and rehabilitation areas, can be identified. Second, a quality of life perspective draws attention to determinants of health at a range of levels, specifically personal factors such as attitudes and beliefs; community factors such as family, peers, employment, and schools; and structural factors such as income distribution, educational opportunities, and employment opportunities. Third, a quality of life perspective can be linked to health promotion and rehabilitation perspectives, suggesting means of promoting positive health and healthy behaviors among adolescents, both well and ill [16]. Finally, a quality of life perspective can identify sensitive adolescent issues that may be affected by illness or disability and the effects of treatments and interventions.

CENTRE FOR HEALTH PROMOTION MODEL

The Ontario (Canada) Ministry of Community and Social Services initially contracted the Centre for Health Promotion, University of Toronto, to develop a model and associated instrumentation to assess the quality of life of persons with developmental disabilities. Quality of life was defined as: "The degree to which a person enjoys the important possibilities of his/her life." The definition can be simplified to "How good is your life for you?" The enjoyment of important possibilities occurs in three domains (see Chapter 3). The philosophic rationale is presented elsewhere [17,18].

Here, the application of this model to adolescents is described. The development of the Quality of Life Profile: Adolescent Version (QOLPAV) is reviewed and findings from an initial validation provided. The reliability of QOLPAV scores and their association with measures of adolescent functioning, health status, and tobacco and alcohol use is described. The relationship of socioeconomic status to adolescents' self-reported quality of life is also examined.

METHOD

Instrument Development

Development of the QOLPAV began with a series of six group meetings with high-school students. Each group consisted of 6–8 volunteers, and groups were held across the range of grade levels (Ontario secondary schools have grades 9–13). Separate meetings with six guidance counselors were held, but generally adolescents' contributions proved more useful. Adolescents were asked: "What does the term 'quality of life' mean to you?" and "What are some areas of concern to adolescents?" Responses were collected, reviewed by the authors, and developed into instrument items. Although all the significant adolescents' contributions were included (determined by whether these issues were raised across at least four of the six groups), some areas not mentioned but suggested by the adolescent development literature were added. The specific adolescent theories drawn on included identity development theory [19], the developmental task approach [20], and socialization theory [21]. The conceptual model suggested avenues as well. Finally, the adolescent health literature was drawn on to identify issues such as alcohol and tobacco use, nutrition, fitness, and sexual knowledge [12]. In most cases, items reflected a combination of sources.

Instrument Description

The QOLPAV consists of 54 items, six in each of nine subdomains. The respondent provides *importance* and *enjoyment* ratings for each item along a five-point scale. In this application, we operationalize the concept of *enjoyment* in terms of personal satisfaction with an aspect of life. (For the remainder of this paper, we therefore refer to satisfaction scores.) In other applications involving nonverbal or disabled groups, enjoyment could be operationalized in slightly different ways, such as attainment in a satisfactory way. The instrument is available from the authors.

SCORING THE QOLPAV

Importance and *satisfaction* scores can range from 1 ("Not at All Important"/"No Satisfaction at All") to 5 ("Extremely Important"/"Extremely Satisfied"). Importance scores serve as a weight for converting satisfaction scores into quality of life (QOL) scores [QOL = (Importance Score / 3) × (Satisfaction Score − 3)]. Items rated as high in importance and satisfaction produce especially high QOL scores. Items rated high in importance and low in satisfaction produce especially low QOL scores. Less importance leads to more moderate quality of life. QOL scores range from −3.33 ("Extremely Important" items, "No Satisfaction at All") to +3.33 ("Extremely Important" items, "Extremely Satisfied"). To illustrate, an individual who describes an item as "very important" (4) with high satisfaction (4) receives a QOL score of 1.33 $[(4 / 3) \times (4 - 3)]$. An individual who rates an item as "not very important" (2) and reports hardly any satisfaction (2) receives a score of $-.67$ $[(2 / 3) \times (2 - 3)]$.

CONTROL AND OPPORTUNITY SCORES

Single items address the amount of control and opportunities the adolescent perceives in each of the nine subdomains. Although these measures are not part of the computation of QOL scores, they provide contextual information within which those scores can be interpreted. The questions are "How much control do I have over ..." and "Are there opportunities for me to improve ... : my physical health; my thoughts and feelings; my beliefs and values; the places where I spend my time; who I spend my time with; being able to use what my community has to offer; the everyday things I can do in my life; the things I can do for fun and enjoyment; and the things I can do to improve myself." *Control* scores can range from 1 (almost no control) to 5 (almost total control), as do *opportunity* scores (almost none ... great many).

Procedure

Study participants consisted of 160 Anglophone students enrolled in a secondary school in the Northern Ontario city of Sudbury. Through arrangements with the secondary school and its teachers, two grade 9 ($n = 45$) classes, two grade 11 ($n = 37$) classes, two grade 12 ($n = 50$) classes, and one grade 13 ($n = 28$) class agreed to participate. Administration was through group self-report by paper-and-pencil completion of the QOLPAV, a number of short validation instruments, and a Personal Characteristics Questionnaire.

Instrumentation

In addition to the QOLPAV, participants responded to three short scales taken from the Youth in Transition Study [22]: a three-item

Satisfaction With Life index (α = .80), six items from the Rosenberg Self-Esteem (α = .85) measure, and a four-item Social Support (α = .78) index. Participants also completed a 10-item Life Chances Questionnaire (α = .70) [23] and an Information About Myself measure, contents of which are provided below (as are from the present administration). Owing to time limitations, short measures that reflected commonly considered adolescent issues were chosen.

To examine whether quality of life is related to the occurrence of healthy behaviors, the tobacco and alcohol use questions from Canada's Health Promotion Survey [24] were asked. Finally, the socioeconomic status of parents using the Blishen socioeconomic index of occupations for Canada was estimated [25]. It is based on amount of education required for, and expected income of, the occupation.

RESULTS

Student Characteristics

Age and gender. Respondents' ranged in age from 14–20 years with a mean of 17.4 years (*SD* = 1.7). The 69 (38%) male and 98 (62%) female students were enrolled in grades 9, 11, 12, and 13. Compared to a national sample of 15- to 19-year-olds [24], a greater proportion of respondents indicated their health as poor (6% versus 1%) or fair (13% versus 6%). Eighteen percent of the present group rated their health as excellent and 63% as good.

Socioeconomic status for each adolescent was taken as the highest of the mother's or father's occupation as scored by the Blishen index. Usable data were obtained from 110 adolescents; mean score was 47.20 (*SD* = 14.22). The scale ranges from 21 (laborer or share cropper) to 101 (physician or dentist).

Seventy-three percent reported having had an alcoholic drink in the last 12 months, somewhat lower than the national average of 80% for 15- to 19-year-olds [26]. However, 38% indicated they smoked cigarettes, a figure much higher than the national average of 19% [27]. Among smokers, the average number of cigarettes smoked daily was 9.5 (*SD* = 6.4).

Importance and Satisfaction

Mean domain and subdomain scores and associated standard deviations for importance and satisfaction are presented in Table 4.1. The subdomains rated as most important were growth becoming, psychological being, and community belonging. Rated somewhat lower in importance was the practical becoming area. Satisfaction was highest for leisure becoming, spiritual being, growth becoming, and social belonging. Somewhat lower satisfaction was seen for community belonging, psychological being, and practical becoming.

Table 4.1: Importance and Satisfaction Scores for the Domains and Subdomains of the QOLPAV

QOL Domain	Importance		Satisfaction	
	Mean	SD	Mean	SD
Being items	4.00	.51	3.62	.60
Physical being	3.97	.64	3.63	.65
Psychological being	4.12	.61	3.47	.70
Spiritual being	3.90	.66	3.77	.67
Belonging items	4.00	.49	3.57	.59
Physical belonging	3.95	.68	3.64	.67
Social belonging	4.01	.56	3.74	.69
Community belonging	4.03	.62	3.32	.76
Becoming items	3.93	.55	3.72	.60
Practical becoming	3.61	.70	3.56	.72
Leisure becoming	3.88	.64	3.84	.71
Growth becoming	4.28	.62	3.74	.69
All items	3.97	.45	3.63	.52

QOL Scores

Quality of life scores were generally positive. Perusal of plots of overall QOL scores revealed that the scores were normally distributed with virtually no skewing. As shown in Table 4.2, QOL scores parallel those seen for satisfaction scores.

Table 4.2: QOL, Control, and Opportunities Scores with Internal Consistencies of QOL Scores

QOL Domain (α for QOL Scores)	QOL		Control		Opportunities	
	Mean	SD	Mean	SD	Mean	SD
Being items (.85)	.97	.80	4.08	.67	3.60	.83
Physical being (.68)	.97	.93	4.05	1.00	3.83	.99
Psychological being (.72)	.78	1.02	3.95	1.13	3.56	1.08
Spiritual being (.71)	1.17	.92	4.25	.83	3.40	1.25
Belonging items (.83)	.87	.81	3.93	.68	3.28	.89
Physical belonging (.67)	.92	.95	4.06	1.02	3.32	1.23
Social belonging (.69)	1.12	.96	4.53	.72	3.49	1.28
Community belonging (.68)	.55	1.03	3.20	1.06	3.03	1.15
Becoming items (.87)	1.13	.80	4.14	.69	3.65	.92
Practical becoming (.74)	.91	.88	4.16	.90	3.64	1.13
Leisure becoming (.74)	1.32	.95	4.20	.86	3.58	1.16
Growth becoming (.79)	1.17	1.02	4.07	.98	3.73	1.04
All items (.94)	.99	.71	4.05	.52	3.51	.74

Control and Opportunities

Greater control was seen for social belonging, spiritual being, and leisure becoming; and the least for community belonging. Adolescents perceived more opportunities in the physical being and growth becoming areas, but somewhat less for community belonging and physical belonging. Subdomains for which control scores were higher showed higher QOL ($r = .79$), as did those subdomains with higher opportunities scores ($r = .53$). Subdomains with higher control ratings had higher opportunities ratings ($r = .58$).

The nine control items, made into a scale, were internally consistent ($α = .70$), as were the nine opportunity items ($α = .83$). Among individuals, overall control scores correlated ($r = .53$) with overall QOL, and opportunities correlated ($r = .15$) with overall QOL scores. Individuals' control and opportunities scores also correlated ($r = .29$).

Reliability of QOL Scores

Cronbach Alpha was calculated for QOL scores for each subdomain, domain, and the overall measure. Internal consistency coefficients for each subdomain were calculated from the six items contained within it, those for each domain from its 18 items, and those for the overall measure from all 54 items. These coefficients are contained in Table 4.2.

The coefficients obtained for the overall measure and for the three broad domains were very promising, exceeding $\alpha = .80$ in every case. Within subdomains, which consist of only six items each, the coefficients were acceptable, being close to or exceeding $\alpha = .70$ in every instance.

Association of QOL Scores with Validation Measures

Quality of life scores were correlated with self-esteem, life satisfaction, social support, and life chances. As seen in Table 4.3, the overall pattern is one of significant correlations of QOL scores across all measures. There was little differentiation among correlations with the various quality of life subdomains. The expected differential correlations of the measures with the specific subdomains of the QOLPAV were not seen.

Table 4.3: Correlations of QOL Scores with Four Validation Measures

QOL Domain	Validation Measures			
	Self-Esteem	Life Satisfaction	Social Support	Life Chances
Being	.53	.50	.45	.44
Physical	.40	.26	.31	.43
Psychological	.51	.50	.40	.36
Spiritual	.42	.49	.42	.33
Belonging	.46	.42	.50	.34
Physical	.32	.29	.32	.24
Social	.46	.46	.52	.35
Community	.36	.29	.40	.24
Becoming	.52	.45	.41	.43
Practical	.49	.41	.40	.39
Leisure	.36	.33	.26	.31
Growth	.48	.44	.37	.37
Overall QOL	.56	.51	.51	.45

Note: All coefficients $p < 0.1$. All tests one-tailed.

Relationship of Quality of Life Scores to Age, Self-reported Health Status, Cigarette Smoking, and Alcohol Use

No differences were seen between males and females for any QOL domain or subdomain scores. Age was related ($p < .05$) to overall QOL scores ($r = -.16$), but not to any of the four validation measures. Age was also related to whether adolescents smoked cigarettes ($r = .27$, $p < .01$), number of cigarettes smoked ($r = .27$, $p < .05$), whether alcohol had been drunk in the last 12 months ($r = .39$, $p < .01$), and frequency of alcohol drinking ($r = .37$, $p < .01$). Since age was related to QOL scores as well as alcohol and tobacco use, the analyses examining correlations of quality of life with alcohol and tobacco use partialled out the effects of age. As health status was not related to age ($r = .06$, ns), correlations with QOL presented in Table 4.4 are not adjusted for age.

As expected, self-reported health status was consistently related to quality of life; and the relationship was especially apparent for the physical being area. Physical being scores were uniquely related to whether an adolescent smoked or not; yet these, and all other QOL scores, were unrelated to the number of cigarettes smoked daily by smokers. Similarly, QOL scores were related to whether an adolescent drank alcohol or not, but not to the frequency of alcohol use.

Table 4.4: Correlation of QOL Scores with Age, Health Status, Tobacco Use, and Alcohol Use

QOL Domain	Age ($n = 155$)	Health Status ($n = 158$)	Tobacco ($n = 158$)	Alcohol ($n = 158$)
Being	-.16*	.34**	-.11	-.25**
Physical	-.15*	.36**	-.27**	-.28**
Psychological	-.15*	.27**	-.03	-.15*
Spiritual	-.10	.23**	-.06	-.21*
Belonging	-.19**	.23**	.02	-.15*
Physical	-.21**	.06	-.01	-.15*
Social	-.12	.24**	.05	-.12
Community	-.13	.27**	.02	-.09
Becoming	-.09	.23**	.03	-.17*
Practical	-.05	.18*	-.05	-.23**
Leisure	-.05	.19**	.03	-.05
Growth	-.11	.19**	.08	-.15*
Overall QOL	-.16*	.30**	-.02	-.21**

Note: Coefficients for cigarette and alcohol use are partial correlations controlling for age. *$p < .05$, **$p < .01$. All tests one-tailed.

Socioeconomic Status and Quality of Life

For QOL, only *psychological being* was related to socioeconomic status ($r = .22$, $p < .05$).

DISCUSSION

QOLPAV scores appeared to be reliable and were related to measures of adolescent functioning, self-reported health status, and tobacco and alcohol use. Expectations of differential subdomain associations with validation measures, however, were generally not met, and relationships with socioeconomic status were weak.

Specific Importance, Satisfaction, and QOL Findings

While developing the QOLPAV, issues identified as important by adolescents, as well as those suggested by the literature, were explored. The validation study provided a more structured opportunity—as part of the scoring of the QOLPAV—to check this process by having adolescents rate each item for importance. The generally high importance ratings provided for the items found in the QOLPAV indicated that its content assessed relevant aspects of these adolescents' lives. The very high importance ratings for items concerned with improvement and change (growth becoming) and thoughts and feelings (psychological being) were consistent with views of adolescence as a period of transition, sometimes involving psychologic distress [19–22].

Psychometric Properties

Domain and subdomain scores were reliable, and quality of life correlated with a range of other indicators of adolescent coping and adjustment. Also, quality of life was related to health status, consistent with the extensive health-related literature [28]. The latter finding suggests the instrument may be sensitive to effects of illness. The relationship with health status was especially high for the being subdomains, providing some evidence of discriminative validity among the subdomain scores.

QOL scores were also related to tobacco and alcohol-related behaviors, but not frequency or intensity of use.

One disappointing finding was the lack of a relationship of QOL scores to socioeconomic status. Based on the determinants of adolescent health literature, it was expected that socioeconomic status would be related to higher QOL scores [12,29]. In our conceptualization of quality of life, environments are expected to play a role, and socioeconomic status was expected to serve as an indirect indicator of environmental quality. Socioeconomic status was also unrelated to alcohol and tobacco use.

It was found, however, that self-perceived control scores as measured by the QOLPAV were related to QOL scores. The correlational nature of this study precludes any conclusion concerning the direction of effects. If these findings are reliable, and personal control could be demonstrated in longitudinal study to be predictive of QOL scores, it would support the increasing importance being ascribed to control as a determinant of health [30,31]. Essentially, however, outside of the relationship of health and control to quality of life, we know little concerning the predictors of QOL scores as measured by the QOLPAV. These need to be explored in further work.

CONCLUSION

Quality of life is an increasingly important focus in health promotion and rehabilitation [16]. The extent to which this particular quality of life perspective and measure will be useful will depend on the congruence of the model's assumptions with those of potential users. We believe that a quality of life perspective can provide insights into the nature and sources of adolescent health. The quality of life of adolescents and its relation to adolescent health may, therefore, be a fertile area of inquiry.

REFERENCES

1.   Dryfoos, J. Adolescents at risk: Prevalence and prevention. New York: Oxford University Press, 1990.

2. Millstein, S.G., Litt, I.F. Adolescent health. In: Feldman, S., Elliot, G. eds. At the threshold: The developing adolescent. Cambridge, MA: Harvard University Press, 1990.

3. Millstein, S.G., Petersen, A.C., Nightingale, E.O., eds. Promoting the health of adolescents: New directions for the twenty-first century. New York: Oxford University Press, 1993.

4. National Research Council: Losing generations: Adolescents in high-risk settings. Report of the Panel on High Risk Youth. Washington, DC: National Academy Press, 1993.

5. Hurrelman, K., Losel, F. Basic issues and problems of health in adolescence. In: Hurrelman K., Losel, F., eds. Health hazards in adolescence. New York: Walter de Gruyter, 1990:1–24.

6. Hechinger, F.M. Fateful choices: Healthy youth for the 21st century. New York: Carnegie Foundation, 1992.

7. Epp, J. Achieving health for all: A framework for health promotion. Ottawa, ON: Health and Welfare Canada, 1986.

8. Pederson, A., O'Neill, M., Rootman, I., eds. Health promotion in Canada. Toronto, ON: W. B. Saunders, 1994.

9. Schabas, R. Opportunities for health. Toronto, ON: Ministry of Health, 1992.

10. U.S. Department of Health and Human Services. Healthy people 2000. Washington DC: U.S. Department of Health and Human Services, 1991.

11. Ontario Ministry of Health. Mandatory health programs and service guidelines. Toronto, ON: Queens Printer, 1989.

12. Raphael, D. The determinants of adolescent health: Evolving definitions, recent findings, and proposed research agenda. Adol Health 1996:19:6–16.

13. Lindstrom, B. Quality of life: A model for evaluating "Health for All." Conceptual considerations and policy implications. Soz Praventivmed 1992;37:301–6.

14. Lindstrom, B. The essence of existence: On the quality of life of children in the Nordic countries. Goteborg, Sweden: The Nordic School of Public Health, 1994.

15. Raphael, D. Quality of life and adolescent health. In: Renwick, R., Brown, I., Nagler, N., eds., Quality of life in health promotion and rehabilitation: Conceptual approaches, issues, and applications. Thousand Oaks, CA: Sage, 1996.

16. Renwick, R., Brown, I., Nagler, N., eds., Quality of life in health promotion and rehabilitation: Conceptual approaches, issues, and applications. Thousand Oaks, CA: Sage, 1996.

17. Raphael, D., Brown, I., Renwick, R., et al. Quality of life theory and assessment: What are the implications for health promotion? Issues in health

promotion monograph series. Toronto, ON: Centre for Health Promotion, University of Toronto and ParticipACTION, 1994.

18. Woodill, G., Renwick, R., Brown, I., Raphael, D. Being, belonging and becoming: An approach to the quality of life of persons with development disabilities. In: Goode, D. ed. Quality of life for persons with disabilities: International issues and perspectives. Boston, MA: Brookline Press, 1994.

19. Erikson, E. Identity, youth and crisis. New York: Norton, 1968.

20. Havighurst, R.J. Human development and education. New York: Longmans, Green, 1953.

21. Elder, G.H Jr. Family structure and socialization. New York: Arno Press, 1980.

22. Bachman, J.G, Kahn, R.L. Mednick, M.T. et al. Youth in transition: Vol. 1: Blueprint for a longitudinal study of adolescent boys. Ann Arbor, MI: Institute for Social Research, University of Michigan, 1967.

23. Jessor, R., Donovan, J.E. Costs F. Perceived life chances, and adolescent health behavior. In: Hurrelman, K., Losel, F., eds., Health hazards in adolescence. New York: Walter de Gruyter, 1990:25–42.

24. Stephens, T., Graham, D., eds. Canada's health promotion survey 1990: Technical report. Ottawa, ON: Minister of Supply and Services, Canada, 1993.

25. Blishen, B.R., Carrol, W.K., Moore, C. The 1981 socioeconomic index for occupations in Canada. Can Rev Sociol Anth 1987;24:465–88.

26. Adlaf, E. Alcohol and other drug use. In: Stephens, T., Graham, D. eds. Canada's health promotion survey 1990: Technical report. Ottawa, ON: Minister of Supply and Services, Canada, 1993:133–24.

27. Pederson, L. Smoking. In: Stephens. T., Graham, D., eds., Canada's health promotion survey 1990: Technical report. Ottawa, ON: Minister of Supply and Services, Canada, 1993:91–102.

28. Stewart, A., Ware, J. Measuring functioning and well-being: The Medical Outcome Study approach. Durham, NC: Duke University Press, 1992.

29. U.S. Office of Technology Assessment. Adolescent health. Washington, DC: U.S. Office of Technology Assessment, 1991.

30. Rodin, J. Health, control, and aging. In: Baltes, M. Baltes, P. eds. The psychology of control and aging. Hillsdale, NJ: Lawrence Erlbaum Associates, 1986.

31. Wallston, B.S., Wallston, K.A., Kaplan, G.D., Maides, S.A., Development and validation of the health locus of control (HLC) scale. J Consult Clin Psychol 1976;44:580–5.

CHAPTER 5

Measuring the Quality of Life of Older Persons

Dennis Raphael, Ivan Brown, Rebecca Renwick, Maureen Cava, Nancy Weir, and Kit Heathcote

OVERVIEW AND PURPOSE

Quality of life (QOL) issues influence the planning, delivery, and evaluation of health and medical services (Renwick et al., 1996). At a minimum, improved QOL is a desired outcome of interventions. QOL assessments can also identify individuals at risk for poor health in the absence of diagnosed illness. And, from a health promotion perspective, QOL assessments can identify interventions that promote health and prevent illness through enhancement of older persons' environments.

We present a new QOL model for older adults that has implications for community and public health nursing. We describe its associated instrumentation and provide evidence concerning its reliability and validity. Applications of the model are presented.

THE CENTRE FOR HEALTH PROMOTION QOL MODEL

We defined QOL as: "The degree to which a person enjoys the important possibilities of his/her life." The enjoyment of important possibilities occurs in three major life domains: *Being, Belonging,* and *Becoming.* These are described in Chapter 3.

INSTRUMENT DEVELOPMENT AND DESCRIPTION

The development of the *Quality of Life Profile: Seniors Version* (QOLPSV) began with a series of 12 group meetings with older persons (age 55+).

These persons were reached through contacts of the North York Public Health Department. Most were involved in health promotion groups carried out in churches, community centres, and activity and cultural groups. These persons were asked: "What does the term 'quality of life' mean to you?" and "What are some areas of concern to seniors?" These comments were collected, reviewed by the authors, and developed into instrument items. While virtually all older persons' contributions were included, some areas were added by service providers (e.g., foot care), and others were suggested by the literature on aging (e.g., vision and hearing issues).

The QOLPSV consists of 111 items: 12 items in each of the first six subdomains and 13 in the last three. The respondent provides *Importance* and *Enjoyment* (the latter operationalized in this application as satisfaction) ratings for each item. Table 5.1 provides examples of items. When making *Importance* and *Enjoyment* ratings, the individual responds to the questions "How important to me is this aspect of my life?" and "How satisfied am I with this aspect of my life?" with either Extremely, Very, Somewhat, Not Very, or Not At All options. Don't Know (DK) or Not Applicable (N/A) responses are allowed.

The respondent also indicates the amount of Control he or she perceives in the broad nine subdomains (Almost Total, Much, Some, Not Much, or Almost None) and Opportunities for change or improvement (Great Many, Many, Some, A Few, Almost None). While these measures are not part of the computation of QOL, they provide information by which these scores are interpreted.

VALIDATION STUDY

The purpose was to: (a) examine the internal consistency reliability of the QOLPSV; (b) evaluate the concurrent validity of the QOLPSV; and (c) examine correlates of QOLPSV scores. Measures chosen to validate the instrument such as the Life Satisfaction and MUNSCH scales were chosen to assess general congruence of QOL with well-being. The Social Health Battery was chosen to assess the specific relationship with aspects of *Social Belonging*. The *Activity* items were chosen to relate specifically to aspects of daily and leisure activities.

Table 5.1: Examples of Items in the QOLPSV

Domain	Item (Respondent Rates Each for Importance and Enjoyment)
Physical Being	Being physically able to get around my home/neighbourhood. Good nutrition and eating the right foods.
Psychological Being	Being able to have clear thoughts. Coping with what life brings.
Spiritual Being	Feeling that my life is accomplishing something. Participating in religious or spiritual activities.
Physical Belonging	Having a space for privacy. Living in a place especially equipped for seniors.
Social Belonging	Being able to count on family members for help. Having neighbours I can turn to.
Community Belonging	Being able to get dental services. Going to places in my neighbourhood (stores, etc.).
Practical Becoming	The caring I do for a spouse or other adult. Doing work around my home (cleaning, cooking, etc.).
Leisure Becoming	Having hobbies (gardening, knitting, painting, etc.). Participating in organized recreation activities.
Growth Becoming	Improving or keeping up my thinking and memory skills. Adjusting to changes in my personal life.

METHOD

Subjects were 205 older persons participating in the North York Public Health Department's Healthful Living Program. Administration involved paper-and-pencil completion of the QOLPSV, one validation instrument, and a demographics questionnaire. It was carried out by 15 public health nurses to 15 groups consisting of, on average, 20 older persons. A total of 205 usable data sets were received (67% response rate). Total administration took 60 minutes: completion of the QOLPSV took from 20 to 40 minutes.

The number completing each measure and the associated internal consistencies, using Cronbach's Alpha, were: Life Satisfaction Scale (Neugarten et al., 1961) [n = 53; α = 0.78]; Memorial University of Newfoundland Scale of Happiness (Kozma et al., 1991) [n = 23; α = 0.94]; Social Health Battery (Donald and Ware, 1984) [n = 35; α = 0.73]; and

National Council on Aging Activity Questionnaire (National Council on the Aging, 1975) [n = 32; α = 0.77].

RESULTS

Demographics

Average age of the respondents was 73 years (SD = 6.97), and of the 199 providing gender information, 46 (23%) were male and 153 (77%) female. Forty-four percent were married, 42% widowed, 6% never married, 3% separated, and 6% divorced. About 40% had not graduated high school, while 34% had at least some college or university education. Ten percent indicated incomes of less than $6,000, while 14% reported annual incomes of $50,000 or higher. The sample was similar in self-reported health status (Excellent, 15%; Very Good, 30%; Good, 29%; Fair, 22%; and Poor, 4%) to the national sample studied in Canada's 1990 Health Promotion Survey (Penning and Chappell, 1993).

Importance, Enjoyment, and QOL Scores

Mean scores and associated standard deviations for the nine sub-domains are presented in Table 5.2. *Importance* and *Enjoyment* scores range from 1 (Not at All Important or Not at All Satisfied) to 5 (Extremely Important or Extremely Satisfied). *QOL Scores* range from −3.33 (Not at All Satisfied with Extremely Important Issues) to +3.33 (Extremely Satisfied with Very Important Issues). A score of >1.50 is considered excellent and scores of 0.51 to 1.50 indicate a very acceptable situation. Scores of −0.50 to +0.50 indicate an adequate situation, scores of −0.51 to −1.50 are problematic, and scores of −1.50 or lower are very problematic.

Table 5.2: Importance, Enjoyment, and Basic QOL Scores for the Nine Subdomains of the QOLPSV (n = 205)

QOL Domain	Importance		Enjoyment		Basic QOL	
	Mean	SD	Mean	SD	Mean	SD
Being	4.28	0.50	3.69	0.69	1.08	1.07
Physical	4.43	0.52	3.71	0.79	1.11	1.23
Psychological	4.35	0.56	3.78	0.76	1.10	1.23
Spiritual	4.05	0.62	3.67	0.70	1.06	1.07
Belonging	4.06	0.55	3.80	0.66	1.19	1.00
Physical	4.22	0.57	4.02	0.67	1.55	1.06
Social	3.87	0.68	3.66	0.71	1.04	1.05
Community	4.07	0.63	3.65	0.75	0.99	1.14
Becoming	3.62	0.62	3.46	0.70	0.77	0.98
Practical	3.39	0.72	3.51	0.76	0.84	1.03
Leisure	3.52	0.75	3.41	0.82	0.74	1.07
Growth	3.92	0.69	3.45	0.75	0.76	1.11
Total Scale	4.00	0.50	3.64	0.63	0.97	0.94

IMPORTANCE SCORES

The *Being* domain was rated the highest, and the *Becoming* domain the lowest. Within the *Being* domain, all subdomains were rated high. Within the *Belonging* domain, *Physical Belonging* was rated the highest and *Social Belonging* somewhat lower. Within the *Becoming* domain, *Growth Becoming* was rated highest. The high ratings across the entire instrument support the view that the QOLPSV captures important components of older persons' QOL.

ENJOYMENT SCORES

Satisfaction with *Belonging* was slightly higher than *Being* and somewhat more than *Becoming* items. Within *Being* and *Becoming*, there was little variation. Within *Belonging*, however, *Physical Belonging*, primarily representing individuals' home environments, was rated higher than other subdomains.

QOL SCORES

These scores paralleled *Enjoyment* scores. *Belonging* scores were generally higher, especially *Physical Belonging*. All three *Belonging* subdomains were <1.

Control and Opportunities

Generally, personal control was seen to exist across domains and subdomains (Table 5.3). The greatest control was seen over *Psychological Being, Social Belonging,* and *Practical Becoming* and least over *Physical Being* and *Community Belonging*. Fewer opportunities for *Practical* and *Leisure* activities were seen.

Table 5.3: Mean Control and Opportunities Scores for the Nine Subdomains of the QOLPSV (n = 205)

QOL Domain	Control		Opportunities	
	Mean	SD	Mean	SD
Being	3.82	0.78	3.58	0.84
Physical	3.65	0.98	3.58	0.97
Psychological	3.96	0.89	3.61	0.94
Spiritual	3.87	0.98	3.59	1.01
Belonging	3.85	0.86	3.55	0.85
Physical	3.91	1.01	3.81	0.97
Social	4.03	0.90	3.52	1.01
Community	3.66	1.04	3.38	1.01
Becoming	3.92	0.83	3.21	1.02
Practical	4.00	0.89	3.17	1.08
Leisure	3.91	0.96	3.16	1.10
Growth	3.87	0.94	3.34	1.18
Total Scale	3.87	0.75	3.45	0.80

Reliability of the QOLPSV

Internal consistency coefficients (Cronbach's α) were calculated for *Importance, Enjoyment,* and *QOL Scores* within each domain and subdomain. All domain and sub-domain indices showed high internal consistency reliability. Cronbach's α for all domain and sub-domain *QOL* scores was >0.90. Alpha for virtually all domain and subdomain *Importance* and *Enjoyment* scores was also >0.90, except for a few instances where values were in the mid 80s. The results of these analyses indicated that all parts of the instrument exceeded common standards of acceptability. The nine *Control* items were also internally consistent ($\alpha = 0.92$), as were the nine *Opportunities* items ($\alpha = 0.92$).

Assessing Validity

The concurrent validity of the QOLPSV was determined through correlations of scores with those obtained from the Life Satisfaction Scale (LSC), Memorial University of Newfoundland Scale of Happiness (MUNSCH), Social Health Battery (SHB), and Activity Items (ACT) taken from the National Council on the Aging (NCA) national survey. While the total sample completed the QOLPSV and the Demographics Questionnaire, only a subsample completed each validation measure. QOLPSV scores can be correlated with each validation measure, but correlating the validation measures with each other was not possible.

The MUNSCH and SHB showed the greatest relationship with overall *QOL* scores (Table 5.4). It was expected that the SHB would be especially related to the *Belonging* domain, and some evidence for this view was seen. Similarly, it was expected that NCA items would show higher correlations with *Becoming* than for other domains and some evidence for this view was also seen. However, in both cases the small sample sizes precluded the assessment of the reliability of these differences. It is difficult to identify differential patterning of scores for the LSS and MUNSCH scores with the specific domains, yet the association of scores with most domains provided beginning evidence of criterion and construct validity.

Table 5.4: Correlation of QOL Scores with the Four Validation Measures

QOL Domains	Validation Measures			
	LSS	MUNSCH	SHB	NCA
Being				
Physical	0.19	0.15	0.45**	0.22
Psychological	0.26*	0.46*	0.47**	0.11
Spiritual	0.22	0.44**	0.46**	0.27
Belonging				
Physical	0.20	0.49*	0.55***	0.38*
Social	0.37*	0.59***	0.57***	0.39*
Community	0.34*	0.62***	0.62***	0.18
Becoming				
Practical	0.30*	0.39*	0.52***	0.36*
Leisure	0.36**	0.36*	0.52***	0.62***
Growth	0.29*	0.47**	0.30*	0.41**
Total Scale	0.37**	0.55**	0.58***	0.42*

*$p<0.05$; **$p<0.01$; ***$p<0.001$

FACTOR ANALYSIS

Our primary focus at this point is upon content validity of our items within domains rather than identifying clusters of older persons' issues. We considered factor analysing QOLPSV item scores. But since there were 111 items and only 205 respondents this analysis would not have met the minimal standards for such a procedure (Harman, 1970) and was not conducted.

Demographic Characteristics and QOL

Self-reported health status was correlated ($p<0.001$) with all sub-domain and total QOL as follows: *Physical Being* (0.57); *Psychological Being* (0.47): *Spiritual Being* (0.39); *Physical Belonging* (0.38): *Social Belonging* (0.37); *Community Belonging* (0.49): *Practical Becoming* (0.38); *Leisure Becoming* (0.42): and *Growth Becoming* (0.40). Health status correlated 0.50 with total *QOL* score. Age was related only to *Physical Being* ($r = -0.16$, $p<0.05$). Finally, education level and reported income were unrelated to all sub-domain scores.

Relationship of Control and Opportunities to QOL

A final analysis examined the relationship of aggregate *Control* and aggregate *Opportunities* scores to QOL. Aggregate *Control* and *Opportunities* showed strong significant ($p<0.001$) correlations (>0.60 and >0.50 respectively) with all domain and subdomain QOL scores.

DISCUSSION

The results indicated that the QOLPSV showed promising psychometric characteristics. QOLPSV scores were related to other measures of positive functioning. QOL was strongly related to happiness as measured by the MUNSCH and social health was strongly related to all QOL subdomains. Further analyses of these patterns were limited by the matrix sampling procedure—necessitated by concern over task demands upon our older persons' sample—and associated small sample size for the validation instruments.

The strong relationship between health status and QOL highlights the importance of promoting means of coping with poor health. The findings concerning the strong relationship between aggregate *Control* and *Opportunities* scores and QOL illustrates their importance and supports (Rodin, 1986a, 1986b) the centrality of control issues among older persons.

Potential Applications of a QOL Focus

The extent to which the QOLPSV will prove useful for those who work with older persons will be a function of the congruence of our model with the assumptions of potential users. One application of a QOL assessment is to use it directly in determining health and service needs. For example, low group scores in a specific QOL domain or sub-domain can suggest priority areas to be addressed in ongoing health programs. On the other hand, the relatively high scores of other items in any assessment would suggest that while these areas should probably not be ignored by social service or health care professionals, there may be less need for focus.

Another application of a QOL perspective is to use it to evaluate the impact of programs, treatments, or other interventions. QOL assessments may be an appropriate and important way to evaluate whether programs have made a difference. A QOL approach can be used for informal assessment of older persons' health needs. This could occur through discussion and review by older persons and health providers of the content in the QOLPSV, or through probability surveys of older persons within a particular area or jurisdiction. The QOLPSV can probably be administered in an interview format, either through face-to-face administration or through telephone surveys. Finally, the QOLPSV can be used in community development activities where review and discussion, as well as application of the QOLPSV by older persons, to older persons, can take place within their communities.

REFERENCES

Donald, C. A., & Ware, J. E. (1984). The measurement of social support. *Research in Community Mental Health, 4*, 325–370.

Harman, H. (1970). *Modern factor analysis.* Chicago, IL: University of Chicago Press.

Kozma, A., Stones, M. J., & McNeil, J. (1991). *Psychological well-being in later life.* Toronto, ON: Butterworths.

National Council on the Aging. (1975). *Codebook for the 'myth and reality of aging'.* Durham, NC: Duke University Center for the Study of Aging.

Neugarten, B., Havighurst, R., & Tobin, S. (1961). The measurement of life satisfaction. *Journal of Gerontology, 16*, 134–143.

Penning, M., & Chappell, N. (1993). Age-related differences. In T. Stephens & D. Graham (Eds.), *Canada's health promotion survey 1990: Technical report* (pp. 247–262). Ottawa, ON: Minister of Supply and Services.

Renwick, R., Brown, I., & Nagler, M. (Eds.) (1996). *Quality of life in health promotion and rehabilitation: Conceptual approaches, issues, and applications.* Thousand Oaks, CA: Sage.

Rodin, J. (1986a). Aging and health: Effects of the sense of control. *Science, 233*, 1271–1276.

Rodin, J. (1986b). Health, control, and aging. In M. Baltes & P. Baltes (Eds.), *The psychology of control and aging* (pp. 139–166). Hillsdale, NJ: Lawrence Erlbaum Associates.

RECOMMENDED READINGS

1. Brown, I., & Brown, R. (2003). *Quality of life and disability: An approach for community practitioners.* New York: Jessica Kingsley Publishers.

   The authors examine the historical context of the concept of quality of life, and discuss the application of quality of life in the daily lives of people who are disabled. Using recent studies to show how the development of quality of life models has led to changes in rehabilitation, and how an understanding of the issue can inform practice in assessment, intervention, management, and policy, this book will be useful to practitioners and managers working with people with disabilities.

2. Canadian Public Health Association. (1996). *Action statement for health promotion in Canada.* Ottawa, ON: Canadian Public Health Association.

   This statement represents an elaboration of the vision provided in the Epp Report (see next). Its three priority action areas are advocating for healthy public policy, strengthening communities, and reforming health systems. The statement is especially noteworthy for its view that "Policies shape how money, power and material resources flow through society and therefore affect the determinants of health. Advocating healthy public policies is the most important strategy we can use to act on the determinants of health."

3. Epp, J. (1986). *Achieving health for all: A framework for health promotion.* Ottawa, ON: Health and Welfare Canada.

   This government document outlines reducing inequities between income groups as an important goal of government policy. It takes a structural approach to health promotion and argues that this would be accomplished by implementing policies in support of health in the areas of income security, employment, education, housing, business, agriculture, transportation, justice, and technology, among others. Arguably, it represents the high-water mark of health promotion in Canada.

4. Fayers, P., & Machin, D. (2007). *Quality of life: The assessment, analysis and interpretation of patient-reported outcomes,* 2nd ed. New York: Wiley.

   This book is an excellent resource on health-related quality of life. Primarily concerned with the outcomes of medical treatment, it is of particular relevance for health care practitioners and clinical and biomedical researchers. The approach is the dominant one among quality of life researchers.

5. Lindstrom, B. (1992). Quality of life: A model for evaluating "Health for All." *Soz Praventivmed, 37,* 301–306.

   The author argues that the potential of the quality of life concept lies in its basically positive meaning and interdisciplinary acceptance. This paper is especially relevant for public health researchers and workers who are trying to communicate a broader view of quality of life than that seen in the clinically oriented health-related area. The article synthesizes a theoretical framework of quality of life that has proven useful for evaluating the health resources of a population.

6. Nussbaum, M., & Sen, A. (2003). *The quality of life*. New York: Clarendon.

The contributors examine how quality of life is central to economic and social assessment and important for public policy, social legislation, and community programs. This collection of essays includes examinations of recent attempts to apply the concept to important practical problems, such as correcting gender-based inequalities, determining medical priorities, and promoting living standards.

7. O'Neill, M., Pederson, A., Dupéré, S., & Rootman, I. (Eds.). (2007). *Health promotion in Canada: Critical perspectives*, 2nd ed. Toronto, ON: Canadian Scholars' Press Inc.

The first edition of *Health Promotion in Canada* was published in the mid-1990s and had a huge impact both in Canada and internationally. The second edition is thematically divided into six key parts—conceptual, national, provincial, international, and practical perspectives, and concluding thoughts—and provides a comprehensive profile of the history and evolution of health promotion in Canada.

8. Poland, B. Health promotion in Canada: Perspectives and future prospects. *Revista Brasileira em Promoção da Saúde, 20*(1), 3–11.

This thoughtful review of the state of health promotion in Canada provides a history of health promotion in Canada. The author then describes the successes and failures of health promotion as well as the reasons and the meaning of these for the future of health promotion in Canada.

9. Renwick, R., Brown, I. & Nagler, M. (Eds.) (1996). *Quality of life in health promotion and rehabilitation: Conceptual approaches, issues, and applications*. Thousand Oaks, CA: Sage.

This contributed book shows how quality of life provides a link between health promotion and rehabilitation. The contributors first review the conceptual basis for understanding and discussing quality of life in health promotion and education. They then address critical issues such as ethics, policy, quality assurance, and measurement—exploring applications of quality of life in the context of a wide range of current social issues and populations.

10. Restrepo, H. E. (2000). *Health promotion: An anthology*. Washington, DC: Pan American Health Organization.

This is a collection of 26 landmark papers that shaped the concept and practice of health promotion. Part I traces the progress of ideas that took root in the 1820s and eventually culminated in the Ottawa Charter for Health Promotion in 1986. "Building healthy public policy" provides the focus for part II, while part III focuses on the challenge of transforming written policy into successful programs. Part IV addresses the development of personal health skills and examines strategies that help people adopt healthy behaviours, while part V focuses on health promotion for specific groups.

RECOMMENDED WEBSITES

1. ACT Health Promotion—www.healthpromotion.act.gov.au

   The ACT Health Promotion website aims to provide professional online information, resources, and support for health promotion workers and all people involved in health promotion practice in the Australian Capital Territory. The introductory URL provided here provides basic information, background, and definitions about health promotion. Especially useful are the glossary of common terms, the brief history, and the links to key health promotion documents.

2. The Atlas of Canada, Quality of Life— http://atlas.nrcan.gc.ca/site/english/maps/peopleandsociety/QOL

   This Government of Canada website assesses quality of life by using indicators of important aspects of a person's life (called domains). It provides indicators categorized into three broad groups: social environment, economic environment, and physical environment. The indicator data generate three quality of life maps for each environment, which are then combined in a fourth map to show overall quality of life. A fifth map, prepared in partnership with the Canadian Policy Research Networks' Quality of Life Indicators Project, shows various national indicators of quality of life.

3. Health Nexus—www.healthnexus.ca

   Health Nexus (formerly the Ontario Prevention Clearinghouse) works to enable communities to promote health in Ontario and beyond. It provides support to organizations and individuals attempting to develop and implement prevention and health promotion strategies. Its three strategic areas of focus are early child development, chronic disease prevention, and health equity (inclusion).

4. Health Promotion 101 On-Line Course—www.ohprs.ca/hp101

   The Ontario Health Promotion Resource System (OHPRS) developed this free course, "Health Promotion 101," as a collaborative effort between its

22 member organizations and with funding from the Ontario Ministry of Health and Long Term Care. OHPRS' role is to support health promoters in Ontario. Health promoters are defined as those who work to promote health, as defined in the Ottawa Charter, in organizations from any sector.

5. The International Society for Quality of Life Research—www.isoqol.org

   The mission statement of this society is: "To advance the scientific study of health-related quality of life and other patient-centered outcomes to identify effective interventions, enhance the quality of health care and promote the health of populations." The society's journal, *Quality of Life Research*, publishes mainly clinically oriented studies.

6. International Union for Health Promotion and Education—www.iuhpe.org

   The International Union for Health Promotion is the only global organization entirely devoted to advancing public health through health promotion and health education. It publishes the journal *Global Health Promotion*, and its members range from government bodies to universities, institutes, non-governmental organizations, and individuals from across all continents.

7. Quality of Life Research Unit—www.utoronto.ca/qol

   The Quality of Life Research Unit has been developing conceptual models and instruments for research, evaluation, and assessment since 1991. In partnership with the Department of Occupational Therapy and Centre for Health Promotion at the University of Toronto, the unit carries out quality of life research that relates to communities, families, and individuals from a variety of population groups. Instruments, reports, manuals, and other publications developed through its research are made available on a cost-recovery basis.

8. *Social Indicators Research*—www.springerlink.com/content/102994

   Social Indicators Research is the leading journal for the publication of research results dealing with the measurement of quality of life. These studies—empirical, philosophical, and methodological—encompass the whole spectrum of society, including the individual, public and private organizations, and municipal, country, regional, national, and international systems. Topics covered include health, population, shelter, transportation, the natural environment, social customs and morality, mental health, law enforcement, politics, education, religion, the media and the arts, science and technology, economics, poverty, and welfare.

9. United Nations Human Development Reports—http://hdr.undp.org/en/statistics

   These reports provide detailed overviews of a number of quality of life indicators on a global basis. They are based on the United Nations' mission of creating an environment in which people can develop their full potential and lead productive, creative lives in accord with their needs and interests. Development is seen as expanding the choices people have to lead lives that they value.

10. World Health Organization Regional Office for Europe: Healthy Cities and Urban Governance—www.euro.who.int/healthy-cities/newsarchive

Based on health promotion principles, the Healthy Cities approach seeks to put health high on the political and social agendas of cities and to build a strong movement for public health at the local level. The concept is underpinned by the principles of the Health for All strategy and Local Agenda 21. Strong emphasis is given to equity, participatory governance and solidarity, intersectoral collaboration, and action to address the determinants of health.

Part II: Community and Policy Perspectives

Part II extends the presentation of quality of life (QOL) approaches from the individual to the community and policy levels. QOL is determined in large part by the environments to which individuals are exposed. These environments come about as a result of public policy decisions made by governments on how to allocate resources. These decisions are frequently influenced by the ideologies and beliefs of members of the governing political parties.

Chapter 6 details how the Centre for Health Promotion's QOL model has been used to examine community QOL. A community-based approach was developed that would allow community members, service providers, and elected representatives to identify the features of a health-promoting community. The role played by public policy in creating such neighbourhood features is examined, as are the barriers to attaining these features.

Chapter 7 applies the community QOL approach to contrast two low-income community members' perceptions of community QOL. Key differences among these neighbourhoods are identified, and much of this has to do with the mix of community members, the social infrastructure that is available to community members, and the political allegiances of the locally elected representatives.

Chapter 8 shows how QOL can be extended to an analysis of public policies in the service of health. Findings from a national study of seniors' QOL in seven cities are presented. Findings of what makes for a good QOL for seniors were remarkably consistent across these cities, as were perceptions of how governments were supporting QOL. For the most part, governments were seen as failing to address many issues of importance to older Canadians.

Chapter 9 places QOL issues within a broad welfare state perspective. Applying the Canadian Policy Research Network's QOL framework, women's QOL in Canada was compared to that in Denmark, the UK, the USA, and Sweden. Indicators of women's QOL are profoundly influenced by the extent to which national governments intervene to provide childcare, employment training, and other supports to their citizens.

CHAPTER 6

Making the Links between Community Structure and Individual Well-being

Dennis Raphael, Rebecca Renwick, Ivan Brown, Brenda Steinmetz, Hersh Sehdevc, and Sherry Phillips

OVERVIEW AND PURPOSE

There is increasing interest in the role that community structures play in promoting health and well-being among citizens (Boutilier et al., 2000; Raphael, 1999; Robert, 1999). These community structures may involve local services (Acheson, 1998); the presence of affordable housing, healthy food, and public transportation (Marmot and Wilkinson, 1999; Wilkinson and Marmot, 1998); community activities that support quality of life (Renwick and Brown, 1996); or the sense of social cohesion that exists among community members (Wilkinson, 1996). Attention is also being paid to how political decision-making supports or hinders the establishment and maintenance of these potentially health-enhancing community structures (Coburn, 2000; de Leeuw, 2000; Teeple, 2000).

The community quality of life approach was developed to elicit community members' understandings of how community aspects either support or do not support health. This approach takes a critical social science perspective that recognizes the complex dialectic between social structure and individual understandings (Eakin et al., 1996; Fay, 1987). This view recognizes that social structures that have the potential to affect health exist within a material world.

The study described here was carried out in collaboration with a number of community agencies in a downtown Toronto neighbourhood (Raphael et al., 1999). The conduct of the study was informed by a model of quality of life previously developed by the first three authors, World Health Organization (WHO) concepts of health, and elements of naturalistic inquiry.

Quality of Life Model

The community quality of life approach focuses on the understandings of community members of what makes life good or not good for them. The quality of life model directs attention to how these factors affect individuals' lives by considering whether and how basic human needs are being met within a community.

Table 6.1 describes the nine domains of quality of life. This model serves as a means of understanding how community factors influence health and well-being.

Table 6.1: Centre for Health Promotion Quality of Life Domains

Physical being	Physical health, mobility, nutrition, fitness, and appearance
Psychological being	Independence, autonomy, self-acceptance, and freedom from stress
Spiritual being	Personal values and standards, and spiritual beliefs
Physical belonging	Physical aspects of the immediate environment
Social belonging	Relationships with family, friends, and acquaintances
Community belonging	Availability of societal resources and services
Practical becoming	Home, school, and work activities
Leisure becoming	Indoor and outdoor activities, and recreational resources
Growth becoming	Learning things, improving skills and relationships, and adapting

WORLD HEALTH ORGANIZATION CONCEPTS OF HEALTH

WHO (1986) defines health as the ability to have and reach goals, meet personal needs, and cope with everyday life. Health is supported by the presence and support by environments of physical, social, and psychological capacities. The WHO framework emphasises the broader or non-medical determinants of health. The Ottawa Charter for Health Promotion (WHO, 1986) outlines peace, shelter, education, food, income, a sound environment, and social justice as necessary for health. These determinants also provided a template against which findings could be considered.

Naturalistic Approach

It was postulated that community quality of life would best be understood by seeing it through the eyes of community members by using a naturalistic approach (Bryman, 1988; Lincoln, 1995; Lincoln and Guba, 1985). Community quality of life is seen as consisting primarily of the understandings and meanings individuals assign to community features.

METHODOLOGY

Community quality of life, therefore, is the concept used to explore factors seen by participants as influencing health. In research communications, such as letters of invitation and introductions to data gathering, the following was stated:

> Being healthy involves more than avoiding being ill. Being healthy is being able to cope with life. We are interested in community and neighbourhood factors which affect health. (Raphael et al., 1998a, p. 43)

Selection of Site

Six Toronto communities served by community health centres (CHCs) were invited to participate in a "study of community quality of life." CHCs serve catchment areas that correspond to geographically well-defined and recognized neighbourhoods.

Two CHCs were chosen on the basis of their contrasting catchment areas and education links with the university and served as the lead collaborating agencies. The two CHC's were the South Riverdale CHC and the Lawrence Heights CHC. In this paper the focus is on the South Riverdale area. Riverdale was chosen as an integrated downtown community with economic and cultural diversity of community members.

Participants

The initial focus in Riverdale was on at-risk groups of seniors, youth, and persons with low income, and the service providers who work with them. As the project evolved, it expanded to include a focus on New Canadians. Elected representatives provided their perceptions of the community. In Riverdale, 14 focus groups involved 102 community members.

There were five groups of adults; three of seniors; three of youth; and three groups of New Canadians. Eleven service providers and six elected representatives were individually interviewed.

Study Process and Questions

Meals were provided for community participants and the usual university ethical protocols of informed consent, voluntary participation, and confidentiality and anonymity were adhered to. Focus group discussions of 45–60 minutes were moderated by the first and fourth authors, and occasionally by other university-based members of the team.

Elected representatives were individually interviewed by university staff and the service providers by university undergraduate students as part of a course requirement. For these 45- to 60-minute interviews, confidentiality and anonymity were not guaranteed, as readers of reports could potentially infer the identity of the contributors.

Community members in the focus groups were asked: *What is it about Riverdale that makes life good for you and the people you care about?* and *What is it about Riverdale that does not make life good for you and the people you care about?*

The complete sets of questions were approved by the members of the Advisory Committee and are available (Raphael et al., 1998b).

FINDINGS FROM THE RIVERDALE STUDY

The Community Context

Riverdale is a downtown community in the eastern section of Toronto. It contains mixed residential, industrial, and commercial/retail areas, with heavy industrial areas in South Riverdale. It is bordered on the west and south by natural features (the Don Valley and Lake Ontario, respectively), on the north by the major Danforth shopping avenue, and on the east by Coxwell Avenue.

With a population of approximately 85,000 people, 20% of whom are of Chinese ancestry, Riverdale is diverse in social class and has a large low-income population and many recent immigrants. There are significant concentrations of Chinese, Greek, and Asians living in areas known as Chinatown, Greektown, and Little India, respectively. As compared to Toronto as a whole, Riverdale, and South Riverdale in particular (where this study was primarily focussed), has a very-low-income population and a high recent immigrant population.

Common Themes Concerning Community Quality of Life

There was striking congruence for some themes across participants (these are reported in Tables 6.2–6.4). Service providers and elected representatives had their own way of seeing the community.

Table 6.2: Community Supports and Barriers to Quality of Life Identified by the Majority of Community Member Groups

Strengths
- Access to food
- Access to amenities
- Churches
- Community activities
- Community agencies and resources
- Diversity of the neighbourhood
- Housing
- Libraries
- Neighbourliness
- Public transportation
- Volunteering at community agencies

Barriers
- Crime and safety
- Cuts to services
- Poverty and unemployment

Table 6.3: Community Supports and Barriers to Quality of Life Identified by the Majority of Service Providers

Supports
Affordable housing
Caring and neighbourly community
Community agencies and resources
Culturally relevant services
Diversity
Public transportation
Barriers
Addictions
Crime and safety
Cuts to services
Environmental issues
Poor housing
Poverty and unemployment

Table 6.4: Community Supports and Barriers to Quality of Life Identified by the Majority of Elected Representatives

Strengths
Access to natural amenities
Community agencies and resources
Cultural diversity
Municipal support for infrastructure
Politically active and caring community
Barriers
Environmental problems
Impact of federal and provincial social policies
Poverty and unemployment

Riverdale Community Quality of Life Model

Based on results from the various focus groups and interviews, a *Riverdale community quality of life model* containing the key elements was developed (Fig. 6.1). The top two ovals represent elements with more macro-level components that are within the domain of government policymaking. Meso-level community components are contained within the next two boxes. These elements concern community institutions that include established services and resources, as well as citizen coalitions and groups. The bottom box contains aspects of the members of the community. Each of these elements are related. Macro-level policies determine in large part the extent to which responsive community institutions are present. These institutions support citizen groups. All of these elements influence the members of the community, who themselves have the potential to influence the higher levels of the model through their activism and support.

The components of the model—and additional community features—are illustrated by quotations from participants in two focus groups that consisted of residents, two service providers, and two elected representatives. Those wishing to examine the comments of other participants can do so by reviewing the write-ups of all of the focus groups and interviews at http://www.utoronto.ca/qol/community.htm.

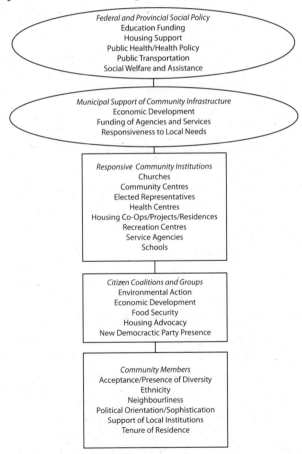

Fig. 6.1: Riverdale community qualify of life model.

Federal and Provincial Social Policy

Federal and provincial policies are seen as having affected the quality of life of community residents. Riverdale has lost many industrial jobs as a result of increasing economic globalization and the shifting of industry that followed in the wake of the North American Free Trade Agreement. These changes have led to increasing economic disparity in the community. In addition to changes in economic conditions, federal and provincial policies—influenced by an agenda of programme reduction and deficit control—have impacted negatively on the most vulnerable of Riverdale residents.

> At the Federal level they're cutting at the foundations. That predisposes provinces to make the cuts they are doing ... The Feds have been very weak in Medicare. They have not been willing to fund what their rhetoric says. (City councillor)

The federal and provincial governments have ended their involvement in social housing, affecting the poor and near poor. More immediately, the Conservative provincial government has cut social services, affecting people with low incomes and, through a ripple effect, local commercial establishments.

Municipal Support of Community Infrastructure

City of Toronto support of local institutions, such as community and recreation centres, is an important component of community quality of life. The City also provides support for local small business through Business Improvement Agencies.

> Jimmy Simpson is a City of Toronto Parks and Recreation Centre. It has a pool, a skating rink, a gym, and a lot of different programs all year round. It is totally funded by the City. The Ralph Thornton Centre is in a city-owned, historic building. We give core administrative funding to that centre and some support for specific programs. We give money for their youth employment programs, their

Chinese seniors programs, and a range of other programs.
(City mayor)

Responsive Community Institutions

Riverdale residents have access to many city-wide supports such as social assistance and public health. There is an extensive network for providing access to food. There also is a range of supportive housing for seniors, those recovering from medical conditions, people with disabilities, and those on low income.

> Food access is one of the major issues that we've identified in this coalition that I'm in, and all of that leading to poor health. The church provides a free community meal ... The volunteers, many of them came first just for the meal, and now they, along with our key lay people, serve the folks who come. (Community minister)

Additionally, Riverdale has a rich network of community-based agencies and services that include recreation and community centres, a CHC, churches, and other organizations. Within these agencies Riverdale residents engage in activities, receive assistance when needed, and work with others to improve the community.

> If you need help in Toronto you can get it but you have to go to the right person or you are lost ... WoodGreen Community Centre is good at Carlaw and Queen. People who work there are very good ... There is the United Church there that can give you help. On health, the welfare system, they can tell me where to get classes, and then it is up to me to go from point A to point B. (Mary, church group)

Citizens' Coalitions and Groups

Riverdale has a tradition of community activism. A number of factors contribute to the rich tradition of citizen activism. The community is economically diverse and its working class background supports a strong New Democratic Party (social democratic) presence. Residents have responded to a series of severe environmental threats and these efforts have been supported by local agencies and elected representatives.

> When I think of Riverdale, I think of activism. People actively involved in trying to make change. It's that mix and that culture of this community that makes life liveable for people here. (CHC program director)

Community Members

Many residents have lived in Riverdale for many years and have developed strong links with other residents and the local agencies.

> I fell once and people stopped and helped me. It was a cold winter day and people called the ambulance. This is when you find out about the little things that neighbours will do for you ... People return a smile. (Helen, church group)

Physical Infrastructure

Riverdale has lots of parks. It is near natural amenities such as Lake Ontario and the Beach area, a natural valley at the western border of the community, and the Leslie Street Spit, a created nature reserve.

> It has some really good natural amenities. It has the Don Valley. It has good parks. It has access to the lake through Cherry Beach, and the Leslie Spit gives access to people to an urban wilderness which is quite noteworthy in North America. (City councillor)

Responsive and Community-oriented Elected Representatives

The political representatives were knowledgeable about Riverdale, its people, its places, and its problems. These elected representatives also understand forces that act upon communities, such as globalization and policy changes, and the challenges faced by those who may be unemployed, of low income, or marginalized or isolated.

> I went to this fellow, told him the problem, and he went to City Hall and got help. It was as simple as picking up a phone. (Helen, church group)

COMMUNITY PROBLEMS

There are environmental problems involving bad air and water.

> We have major problems with landfill sites. Down by the Commissioners (plant) and the torn-down gas stations, there are landfills with animals, sewage, and PCBs. Crummy houses were built on land sites. Industrial stuff that was dumped there [is] coming up. (Mary, church group)

There are ongoing problems of poverty and unemployment. This has been worsened by the Free Trade Agreement with the United States and the North American Free Trade Agreement.

> It used to be a very solid working-class area with a lot of jobs. There were factories and plants in the area, but many of those have closed. (City mayor)

Finally, there are safety and security issues related to crime, vandalism, and personal safety.

> Vandalism still goes around, young kids break the antennae on the cars. It's primarily by youth, at schools and at the recreation centres. Young kids break in, break the locks at the recreation centre. (Mary, church group)

Interestingly, it has been the presence of these problems, and community responses to them, that has contributed to what many people see as the good community quality of life in Riverdale.

DISCUSSION AND RELATIONSHIP TO OTHER LITERATURES

One striking result of the study was the complexity of findings concerning community features seen as influencing health and well-being. Community quality of life is seen as consisting of a very wide range of interacting factors that reflect the unique history of a community. In the case of Riverdale, issues were raised ranging from macro-level political and economic factors, local service and charitable organizations, to the personal characteristics of local residents.

Relationship to the Healthy Cities Concept

The WHO Healthy Cities office in Copenhagen identifies municipal support of social infrastructure and social programs as essential for community health (WHO, 1995). The findings of the perceived importance of social infrastructure, including social and community services, educational opportunities, and employment opportunities, are consistent with the basic core principle of the Healthy Cities movement, derived from a decade of work in European cities.

Threats to the Welfare State

The findings of this study that weakening social infrastructure is seen as threatening health is consistent with the growing literature indicating that societies with extensive services and strong social safety nets show stronger population health (Bartley et al., 1997; Kawachi and Kennedy, 1997). Coburn (2000) has considered how the governing ideology of neo-liberalism may be responsible for weakening social cohesion, social capital, and population health.

CONCLUSION

The presence of community supports and the structures, activities, and outcomes that are seen as accruing from them are the reasons why Riverdale, despite its problems, continues to be a community where people wish to live, rather than leave. Returning to the quality of life model presented in Table 6.1, it is possible to consider how the features of the community of Riverdale support quality of life in the nine domains outlined.

The complexity of the model allows community workers to decide at which level they wish to intervene to improve community quality of life. Workers can continue to use local agencies to support the development of social supports and community cohesion, focus upon policy issues related to funding of services, or help improve access to the natural amenities of Riverdale—among any number of possible interventions.

REFERENCES

Acheson, D., 1998. Independent Inquiry into Inequalities in Health. Stationary Office, London, UK.

Bartley, M., Blane, D., Montgomery, S., 1997. Health and the life course: Why safety nets matter. British Medical Journal 314, 1194–1196.

Boutilier, M., Cleverly, S., Labonte, R., 2000. Community as a setting for health promotion. In: Poland, B., Green, L., Rootman, I. (Eds.), Settings for Health Promotion: Linking Theory and Practice. Sage, Newbury Park, CA, pp. 250–279.

Bryman, A., 1988. Quantity and quality in social research. Unwin Hyman, Boston.

Coburn, D., 2000. Income inequality, lowered social cohesion, and the poorer health status of populations: the role of neo-liberalism. Social Science and Medicine 51, 135–146.

de Leeuw, E., 2000. Beyond community action: Communication arrangements and policy networks. In: Poland, B., Green, L., Rootman, I. (Eds.). Settings for Health Promotion: Linking Theory and Practice. Sage, Newbury Park, CA, pp. 287–300.

Eakin, J., Robertson, A., Poland, B., Coburn, D., Edwards, R., 1996. Towards a critical social science perspective on health promotion research. Health Promotion International 11, 157–165.

Fay, B., 1987. Critical Social Science: Liberation and its Limits. Cornell University Press, Ithaca.

Kawachi, I., Kennedy, B. P., 1997. Health and social cohesion: Why care about income inequality? British Medical Journal 314, 1037–1040.

Lincoln, Y. S., 1995. Emerging criteria for quality in qualitative and interpretive research. Qualitative Inquiry 1, 275–289.

Lincoln, Y. S., Guba, E. G., 1985. Naturalistic Inquiry. Sage, Newbury Park, CA.

Marmot, M. G., Wilkinson, R. G. (Eds.), 1999. Social Determinants of Health. Oxford University Press, Oxford.

Raphael, D., 1999. Health effects of economic inequality. Canadian Review of Social Policy 44, 25–40.

Raphael, D., Steinmetz, B., Renwick, R., 1998a. How to Carry Out a Community Quality of Life Project. A Manual. Department of Public Health Sciences, Toronto.

Raphael, D., Steinmetz, B., Renwick, R., 1998b. The People, Places, and Priorities of Riverdale: Findings from the Community Quality of Life Project. Centre for Health Promotion, Toronto. Available on-line at http://www.utoronto.ca/qol/communit.htm.

Raphael, D., Steinmetz, B., Renwick, Smith, T., Phillips, S., Sehdev, H., 1999. The community quality of life project: A health promotion approach to understanding communities. Health Promotion International 86, 197–207.

Renwick, R., Brown, I., 1996. Being, belonging, becoming: The Centre for Health Promotion model of quality of life. In: Renwick, R., Brown, I., Nagler, M. (Eds.), Quality of Life in Health Promotion and Rehabilitation: Conceptual Approaches, Issues, and Applications. Sage, Thousand Oaks, CA.

Robert, S. A., 1999. Socioeconomic position and health: The independent contribution of community socioeconomic context. Annual Review of Sociology, 489–516.

Teeple, G., 2000. Globalization and the Decline of Social Reform, 2nd ed. Garamond Press, Toronto.

Wilkinson, R. G., 1996. Unhealthy Societies: The Afflictions of Inequality. Routledge, New York.

Wilkinson, R. G., Marmot, M., 1998. Social Determinants of Health: The Solid Facts. World Health Organization, Copenhagen.

World Health Organization, 1986. Ottawa Charter for Health Promotion. Author, Geneva.

World Health Organization, 1995. Twenty Steps for Developing a Healthy Cities Project. WHO Regional Offices, Copenhagen.

CHAPTER 7

Community Quality of Life in Low-income Neighbourhoods

Dennis Raphael, Rebecca Renwick, Ivan Brown, Sherry Phillips, Hersh Sehdev, and Brenda Steinmetz

OVERVIEW AND PURPOSE

There is increasing interest in the role that community structures play in promoting health and well-being among citizens (Boutilier, Cleverly, & Labonte, 2000; Raphael, 1999; Robert, 1999). These community structures may involve local services (Acheson, 1998); the presence of affordable housing, healthy food, and public transportation (Marmot & Wilkinson, 1999; Wilkinson & Marmot, 1998); community activities that support quality of life (Renwick & Brown, 1996); or the sense of social cohesion that exists among community members (Wilkinson, 1996). Attention is also being paid to how political decision-making supports or hinders the establishment and maintenance of these health-enhancing community structures (Coburn, 2000; de Leeuw, 2000; Teeple, 2000). Much of this interest, including the research reported here, has been driven by theoretical work on the social determinants of health as well as the importance of lay perceptions of these social determinants of health.

The community quality of life approach, therefore, is a process by which community features that influence well-being can be identified with the objective of improving them. This paper illustrates the approach by presenting detailed findings from a study of one low-income community. It then considers whether these factors were common to those identified in another Toronto low-income community. Finally, it explores the value of the approach for community developers. The study described here was one of two carried out as a collaboration among community agencies and the University of Toronto.

SELECTION OF NEIGHBOURHOODS

To illuminate community factors seen as influencing health and well-being in low-income neighbourhoods, two very different settings were selected. The key differences are presented in Table 7.1.

Table 7.1: Characteristics of Selected Neighbourhoods

Characteristic	Lawrence Heights	South Riverdale
Municipality	Suburban North York	Urban Toronto
Services/agencies	Limited	Plentiful
Economic diversity	Homogeneous	Heterogeneous
Cultural diversity	Very mixed	White/Chinese
Physical setting	Isolated	Integrated
Political representation	Liberal (traditional capitalist)	New Democratic (social democratic)

Lawrence Heights is a culturally diverse low-income neighbourhood located in suburban north Toronto. Its population of 7,000–8,000 live in rent-geared-to-income public housing in low-rise apartment buildings, townhouses, and single-family homes. It was, at one time, physically cut off from the neighbouring middle-class area by a large wire fence that encircled the neighbourhood. Large sections of the fence have been removed, yet the area remains isolated from other neighbourhoods, with only four roadways leading in and out of it.

Twenty-five years ago, most residents were of European descent and spoke English as their first language. Many had moved to Ontario from other parts of Canada, seeking jobs. Most families had two parents. No services were located within the community. Among those now living in Lawrence Heights, there is a higher than average percentage of women, children, and youth, sole-parent families, seniors, and people who are unemployed than in the Toronto area as a whole. The community has become more culturally and linguistically diverse. Some of the original residents remain, but many have recently come from the Caribbean, Latin America, South Asia, and East Africa. There are businesses in the general area now, although none operate in Lawrence Heights itself. Public and Catholic schools, a community recreation center, a library, and local offices of several social services organizations are now in the immediate area. A large shopping mall is within walking distance. Chapter 6 provides a description of South Riverdale, the other community studied.

METHODOLOGY

Participants in the Lawrence Heights Study

Lawrence Heights' children, youth, adults, and seniors, service providers including teachers within the community, and local elected representatives provided insights on the quality of life. Almost all of the adult groups included New Canadians. The 18 community focus groups involved 146 community members in eight groups of adults, three groups of seniors, and seven groups of children and youth. Twelve service providers and six elected representatives were individually interviewed (using the methods described in Chapter 6).

THE STRUCTURE AND CONTENT OF COMMUNITY QUALITY OF LIFE IN LAWRENCE HEIGHTS

Community features supporting quality of life converged among the study groups. But since groups expressed their perceptions in somewhat different ways and community workers could be working with specific age groups, results are presented by respondent group.

Children and Youth's Perceptions of Community Quality of Life

There was much agreement about community factors that support quality of life. There were some differences, however, between white and non-white participants and between children and youth.

Access to amenities. Having access to shopping and things to do was seen as an important aspect of neighbourhoods. Youth appreciated the nearby mall, yet wished for more variety and input as to what was available there.

Community health centre. The two groups consisting of primarily African-Canadian youth spoke highly of the centre. They saw its value for people of different cultures and provision of help with a range of problems in addition to providing medical care.

Leisure and recreation activities. The most consistent finding from the youth and children groups was the importance of leisure and recreation activities. Having things to do is an important concern. Recreation centres are important because they provide a range of activities, such as clubs, athletics, and social events.

Neighbourliness. Almost all groups felt people within the community care about and help each other. In most cases youth were positive about their neighbours, but the children's groups were less so. Many concrete instances of helping behaviour as well as ideas about cultural solidarity and commitment were provided.

Parkland and open space. The presence of open areas, trees, and parks was a positive aspect of the community. Youth were more positive about this than were children.

Public transportation. Public transportation was an important aspect of the area for all youth groups—it was not raised by the children's groups. While the subway was spoken of positively, there was criticism of the bus service and concern about service cutbacks.

Schools and education. Many positive points were raised about schools and education. Education was important for getting ahead, and schools provided extracurricular activities. Nonetheless, there were many complaints among the groups of youth about the lack of school facilities and lack of respect by teachers.

Adults' Perceptions of Community Quality of Life

Adults shared many of the perceptions of children and youth, but there was greater dissatisfaction concerning the degree to which these features were present.

Access to amenities. Most of the adult groups spoke of the importance of being near to things. The area was convenient for schools, parks, shopping, and public transportation. However, evening service was a problem as some buses stop running at relatively early hours. Some New Canadian groups reported good access to traditional food delivered from outside the neighbourhood or purchased from local stores.

Community agencies and resources. There was agreement that community agencies and resources provide support and assistance. However, in many cases more services were desired and those available could be improved.

Local schools. Many positive experiences with the local schools were related. The local schools were seen as receptive to newcomers and providing extra help when needed.

Neighbourliness. There was divergence of opinion concerning neighbourliness in the community. Each group spoke of the importance of having people with similar backgrounds and languages in the community. However, groups reported mixed experiences with neighbours. Some experienced assistance from neighbours, but others reported frequent disagreements.

Parkland and recreation activities. Almost all groups identified parkland and recreation activities for children as important. Most groups were happy with the local parks and playgrounds and recreation activities. But some felt there should be more for older children and that little recreation was available during the winter.

Services in own language. All groups spoke of the importance of services being in their own language. However, only one group said that this was the case at present.

Seniors' Perceptions of Community Quality of Life

The two groups for whom English was their first language were generally satisfied with the presence of community factors supporting quality of life. This was not the case with the newly arrived from Latin America group of Spanish-speaking seniors.

Access to amenities. The English-language groups spoke about the local mall and how easy it was to shop. Like the youth, having the mall nearby was a means to meet people and socialize.

Community health centre. All three groups viewed the community health centre positively. It provided health care and supported community activities. It helped people with health and tenants issues and in obtaining benefits. Staff were helpful and friendly.

Community recreation centre. The two English-speaking groups spoke of the importance of the community recreation centre. The centre helped people in the community by providing activities for children, adults, and seniors.

Community involvement and volunteer work. These same groups spoke of involvement as important. Seniors felt happier for being involved and benefited from helping others.

Involvement with the seniors group. The importance of involvement in the group was highlighted. The tenants' group worked on community and housing issues. The recreation group was seen as a great way to see people and have fun. The Hispanic group helped in coping and provided opportunities to meet people and discussions in Spanish.

Neighbourliness. The same two groups were positive about their neighbours and provided examples of mutual aid. The Spanish-speaking group saw some neighbours as having personal problems involving family violence.

Public transportation. The groups spoke of the importance of public transportation. While happy with the subway, cutbacks to evening and weekend bus service made it necessary to have a car or take a taxi at those times. Service providers and elected representatives provided similar views.

PROBLEMS FACING LAWRENCE HEIGHTS

There was congruence across all participant groups about the issues faced by Lawrence Heights residents: low income, lack of services, effects of provincial policies, and concerns about crime and safety. Some issues were more likely to be raised by particular participant groups.

Crime and safety. There was a shared concern about crime and safety among the community groups and teachers. Community members saw the neighbourhood as safe during the day, and less so at night. Teachers were concerned about children's exposure to violence.

Cutbacks to services and lack of services. All of the seniors and one adult group expressed concern about service cuts focused on housing maintenance, libraries, bus services, and community services. For every adult and youth group, lack of services was an issue. Adult groups expressed needs for counseling and recreation services for youth, day care, programs for families, training and ESL classes, and culturally sensitive services. Youth and children identified needs for support and recreation services. Every service provider and most representatives discussed shortages of services.

Housing. Lawrence Heights' housing units are managed by the province and municipality. Maintenance concerns were raised in almost every community member group and by most service providers and representatives.

Isolation of the community/need for redevelopment. For elected politicians, geographical and social isolation from the surrounding community needs to be addressed. All of the representatives spoke of the need for redevelopment of the site.

Low income. Low income was mentioned by every service provider and elected representative. Interestingly, the issue did not arise directly among community members; however, as noted, there was extensive discussion of the need for services.

Provincial policies. Most service providers and every elected representative mentioned provincial policies as a problem. It was mentioned indirectly by community members in terms of cuts to services and deteriorating housing.

Racism and racial tensions. There was discussion of racism, racial discrimination, or racial tension among a youth group, five adult groups, and some service providers. The issue was especially important to non-white adults and African-Canadian youth.

UNDERSTANDING COMMUNITY QUALITY OF LIFE IN LAWRENCE HEIGHTS AND SOUTH RIVERDALE

In our earlier study (using identical methodology) of the downtown Toronto neighbourhood of South Riverdale (see Chapter 6), community members identified access to amenities, caring and concerned people, community agencies, low-cost housing, and public transportation as supporting community quality of life (Raphael et al., 2001). Riverdale service providers and representatives recognized diversity, community agencies and resources, and the presence of culturally relevant food stores and services as strengths. Riverdale was seen as well resourced with community agencies and services. While overall a low-income neighbourhood, residents were economically diverse. Additionally, there was a significant Chinese-speaking population as well as smaller cohesive communities of Greek- and Southeast Asian-descended residents.

South Riverdale was seen as a relatively stable neighborhood where many had developed personal networks and commitments to local institutions. It had a reputation for community activism and had historically been represented by members of the social democratic New Democratic Party at local and provincial levels. Upon the completion of these separate studies, the university-based members of the team drew upon their experiences of the two communities as well as the empirical findings to carry out the following analysis. This analysis should serve as a source of hypotheses to be considered in further research.

Differences in Degree of Common Community Features Influencing Quality of Life

Access to amenities. Clearly, this is an important component of community quality of life for both communities. Lawrence Heights is an isolated low-income community whose most immediate source of amenities is a single large shopping mall. In contrast, in South Riverdale a variety of amenities are present within the immediate community.

Community agencies and resources. Lawrence Heights has limited services and is surrounded by middle-class areas for whom service provision has not been an historical priority. The local city government provides little support for community infrastructure. In contrast, South Riverdale has a wealth of service agencies that have been built up over generations as a result of ongoing community activism and support.

Crime and safety. In both communities crime and safety were concerns. In Lawrence Heights the profile of the problem was higher, with concerns about drugs, guns, and violence. In contrast, South Riverdale residents' concerns were limited to youth break-ins and vandalism.

Low income and poverty. Both communities have higher than average numbers of low-income people. Lawrence Heights, however, is a community in which low income is required for residence. Therefore, there is virtually no mixing of socioeconomic levels among residents, a concern raised by the elected representatives. In South Riverdale, supported housing is scattered throughout the area, allowing residents of differing social classes to live in close proximity—a phenomenon seen as positive by most respondents.

Municipal support of community infrastructure. Municipal support to a community like Lawrence Heights is limited to the local recreation centre and road maintenance. South Riverdale, however, has received City of Toronto support for a range of services, such as settlement services, recreation and public health services, and support of local small businesses.

Neighbourliness. Neighbours were a source of support in Lawrence Heights, but the quality of these relationships was problematic and disagreement existed regarding the benefits of involvement with neighbours. Residents' concern for each other was an important contributor to quality of life in South Riverdale. This concern for others was also institutionalized through the establishment of a range of community resources and supports.

Understanding of causes behind service deterioration. In Lawrence Heights—as in South Riverdale—there was widespread concern among residents about reductions in services, but little overt discussion of the political forces driving these reductions. In contrast, South Riverdale residents were more likely to relate these reductions to federal and provincial policies favoring the well-off at the expense of low-income people. This may be due to most Lawrence Heights representatives being Liberal (a mainstream capitalist party), while most Riverdale representatives were New Democrats (a social democratic party).

Differences in Kind of Community Features Influencing Quality of Life

Citizen activism. Lawrence Heights has had few opportunities for community activism. The Lawrence Heights Alliance is the main activist group in the community, but was rarely mentioned by residents. South Riverdale has a history of citizen activism. The roots lie in its diverse socioeconomic mix, the representation of the community by social democrats, and the significant environmental threats, such as lead and air pollution from smelters, factories, and incinerators, that helped mobilize community action.

Cultural mix and stability. South Riverdale is a predominantly white community with a significant Chinese-Canadian community, and somewhat smaller Greek and Southeast Asian communities. These ethnic communities have established residential stability whereby businesses that provide residents with services, food, and other amenities within their own language have been established. In contrast, Lawrence Heights is much more diverse and residents have not established a stable community. The community itself does not have any businesses that would allow culturally related amenities to be easily available.

Economic diversity. Lawrence Heights is defined by its rent-geared-to-income housing. There is a concentration of people whose lives are affected by relatively low income and limited economic resources. The community is isolated from the more well-off communities around it. South Riverdale presents a mix of socioeconomic status. This diversity allows for greater sensitivity on the part of more well-off residents to the problems of less well-off residents and contributes to the greater degree of community activism.

Housing. As noted, housing in Lawrence Heights is of one kind—rent-geared-to-income. South Riverdale also provides housing in the form of seniors housing, co-ops, and rent-geared-to-income projects. However, South Riverdale also has many single-family dwellings such that there is greater diversity of housing within the community. Little complaints were heard about the subsidized housing available.

Political representation. As noted, Lawrence Heights representatives are predominantly Liberal, while South Riverdale's are New Democrats. This both reflects and contributes to the political orientation held by community members.

Racism. A much greater proportion of Lawrence Heights residents were Canadians of colour. In addition, many of these residents were recently arrived from nations from which immigration has been relatively recent. These individuals were much more likely to report incidents of racism than the single largest minority group in South Riverdale—the Chinese.

CONCLUSION

A lesson learned from these studies is the importance of community resources and services for low-income communities. The incidence of low income and income inequality has been increasing in Canada: this, combined with reductions in services and supports, accelerates this process of social exclusion (Raphael, 1999).

While both communities have a significant proportion of low-income residents, there are many aspects of quality of life related to the structure and layout of South Riverdale that limit this process. The physical integration of low-income people into a diverse community, the provision of social services and supports, and the presence of responsive, community-oriented elected representatives are the key ways in which social exclusion is limited. A comparison of these communities identifies a number of hypotheses that can form the basis of further inquiries into processes of social exclusion and their impact on citizens.

Policymakers and service providers can consider the quality of life approach as a means of considering how community structures can affect the health and well-being of community members. Community partners in the studies have used the findings to: (a) orient new staff and students at local agencies as to the community and its characteristics; (b) provide validation for agency activities addressing key quality of life issues and identify areas of needed focus; and (c) justify the maintenance of community resources and agencies that are threatened with budget cuts.

The complexity of community quality of life allows community workers to decide at which level they wish to intervene to improve community quality of life. Workers can use local agencies to support the development of social supports and community cohesion, focus on policy issues related to funding of services, or help improve the natural amenities that may exist within a community—among any number of possible interventions.

REFERENCES

Acheson, D. 1998. *Independent Inquiry into Inequalities in Health*. Stationary Office: London, UK. On-line at http://www.official-documents.co.uk/document/doh/ih/contents.htm.

Boutilier, M., S. Cleverly, & K. Labonte. 2000. Community as a setting for health promotion. In B. Poland., L. Green, & I. Rootman (eds.). *Settings for Health Promotion: Linking Theory and Practice* (pp. 250–279). Newbury Park, CA: Sage.

Coburn, D. 2000. Income inequality, lowered social cohesion, and the poorer health status of populations: the role of neo-liberalism. *Social Science and Medicine* 51: 135–146.

de Leeuw, E. 2000. Beyond community action: Communication arrangements and policy networks. In B. Poland, L. Green, & I. Rootman (eds.), *Settings for Health Promotion: Linking Theory and Practice* (pp. 287–300). Newbury Park, CA: Sage.

Marmot, M. G., & R. G. Wilkinson (eds.). 1999. *Social Determinants of Health.* Oxford: Oxford University Press.

Raphael, D. 1999. Health effects of economic inequality. *Canadian Review of Social Policy* 44: 25–40.

Raphael, D., R. Renwick, I. Brown, S. Phillips, & H. Sehdev. 2001. Making the links between community structure and individual well-being: community quality of life in Riverdale, Toronto, Canada. *Health and Place* 7(3): 17–34.

Renwick, R., & I. Brown. 1996. Being, belonging, becoming: the Centre for Health Promotion model of quality of life. In R. Renwick, I. Brown, & M. Nagler (eds.), *Quality of Life in Health Promotion and Rehabilitation: Conceptual Approaches, Issues, and Applications* (pp. 75–88). Thousand Oaks, CA: Sage.

Robert, S. A. 1999. Socioeconomic position and health: the independent contribution of community socioeconomic context. *Annual Review of Sociology* (pp. 489–516). Palo Alto: Annual Reviews.

Teeple, G. 2000. *Globalization and the Decline of Social Reform* (2nd ed.). Toronto: Garamond Press.

Wilkinson, R. G. 1996. *Unhealthy Societies: The Afflictions of Inequality.* New York: Routledge.

Wilkinson. R. G., & M. Marmot. 1998. *Social Determinants of Health: The Solid Facts.* Copenhagen: World Health Organization. On-line at http://www.who.dk/healthy-cities.

CHAPTER 8

What Do Canadian Seniors Say Supports Their Quality of Life?

Toba Bryant, Ivan Brown, Tara Cogan, Clemence Dallaire, Sophie Laforest, Patrick McGowan, Dennis Raphael, Lucie Richard, Loraine Thompson, and Joyce Young

INTRODUCTION

The health and well-being of Canadian seniors is an important public health focus in Canada.[1-6] During the International Year of Older Persons (IYOP), a national consortium of seven research groups implemented participatory research projects by which seniors would identify and address the factors seen as influencing their quality of life.

This article has two purposes. The first is to show how the key elements of the project—participatory nature, concern with quality of life, determinants of health perspective, and a policy focus—contributed to the establishment of successful research groups across Canada. The second is to present issues seniors see as influencing their quality of life. Such participatory research projects that address seniors' issues from a policy perspective are rare.

In response to Health Canada's IYOP funding announcement, a committee of Toronto researchers and seniors made inquiries to the Federation of Canadian Municipalities and the Canadian Consortium for Health Promotion Research to identify interested seniors groups and university researchers across Canada. Local projects would be participatory, directed by the seniors themselves, and would address issues related to "quality of life." In the participating cities of Quebec City, Montreal, Ottawa, Toronto, Regina, Vancouver, and Whitehorse, seniors councils associated with municipal governments initiated and carried out the research processes.

These concepts—participatory nature, quality of life, and policy emphasis—made the project attractive to seniors. The determinants of health framework was new to most seniors, but was known to the local university staff whose role was to assist the seniors in doing the research. The objectives of the project were to:

- engage Canadian seniors in a process to identify and address the determinants of health and their effects upon health, thereby improving their health;
- provide local, provincial, and federal municipalities with information to form the basis for policy decisions related to the health and well-being of seniors;
- provide resource materials to allow seniors groups across Canada to carry out a similar process of identifying and acting upon health determinants;
- demonstrate participatory activities involving seniors working together with other sectors as a valuable policy-informing activity;
- evaluate the project, its process, and products.

The full reports from each of the seven participating cities are available online as is the original project proposal.[7] An extensive synthesis report on the national study is also available.[8]

BRIEF OVERVIEW OF CONCEPTS INFORMING THE PROJECT

The project drew upon recent advances in understanding how the health of Canada's seniors is affected by individual, community, and societal factors, or what are termed the determinants of health.[9-11] The project provided a mechanism by which seniors could both learn about these determinants and identify their effects upon their health.

Participatory research approach. Participatory research is about subjects of the research having control over the carrying out of the research.[12] In each locality, a Seniors Coordinating Committee of volunteer seniors was established and had final control over the process and product of the research. Project Coordinators were paid through project funds and hired by the local Seniors Coordinating Committee. University support staff provided support and guidance to the project activities and assisted in technical matters of data analysis and report writing.

Quality of life approach. Quality of life is a holistic construct that views human health and well-being within the contexts of proximal and distal environments.[13] It combines elements of broad societal indicators with the actual lived experience of people.[14] Quality of life also offers the advantage of being understandable to both community members and policymakers and can be seen as a proxy for health and well-being.[15] Quality of life is also being considered in national and local policy environments.[16-18]

Determinants of health approach. One purpose of the project was to assess whether seniors' perceptions of quality of life influences would be consistent with Health Canada's determinants of health (e.g., income and social status, social support networks, education, employment and working conditions, physical and social environments, etc.).[19] Such congruence would indicate these concepts were of value to health promotion work with individuals and communities.[9]

METHOD

In each participating city, a lead seniors group—usually a municipal seniors council—supported by a paid project coordinator, university staff, and municipal partners such as the local health unit or city services staff, organized the project. Most projects had strong local university involvement while others had less or none. Each city formed a Seniors Coordinating Committee that controlled the project and an Advisory Committee consisting of representatives from seniors groups, service sectors, and municipal staff. These working groups adapted the general project design to their specific locality.

In each site, data were collected from seniors, service providers, and governmental staff. This paper reports data obtained from seniors. Each city carried out slightly different procedures using varying theoretical frameworks.

This variation could be seen as problematic. But the nature of participatory research is to allow local adaptation of the research process. In any event, the consistency of findings across locations (see below) suggests that the divergence in question wording and study process was not a major problem. See the Appendix for examples of questions applied.

Group discussions and interviews and the data analysis were usually carried out by professionally trained personnel supporting the projects using commonly accepted qualitative research methods.[20]

The approach taken by the Toronto group was typical. Focus group discussions and interviews were tape-recorded and transcriptions of sessions were prepared.

The transcripts were carefully read by two team members—sometimes seniors, sometimes research staff—and key themes and ideas were identified using coloured pens and markers. The process of categorizing and forming themes was repeated until the best fit between the data and the interpretive themes was achieved. The themes for each group or individual were then written up in the form of a six- to seven-page narrative that identified the themes from the session.

These themes were then reviewed and verified by members of the Seniors Coordinating Committee. In essence, then, the process of theme identification involved a team approach of the project participants. Seniors themselves determined the formats of the reports and the interpretations of findings.

RESULTS

There was agreement across all locations as to the importance to seniors' quality of life of the following: access to information, health care, housing, income security, safety and security, social contacts and networks, and transportation. Participants in most localities also identified issues of ageism of society, having voices heard, promoting healthy lifestyles, and lack of political will as barriers to address key issues. The following section highlights some of the issues on which there was consensus across local projects.

Access to Information

Participants expressed concern about seniors' access to information about available programs and services. Seniors need to be able to access information about the availability of services and resources in formats that are easy to read and comprehend. Community organizations and governments must work with seniors to develop and make these kinds of information available. Table 8.1 provides an example that illustrates seniors' concerns over these issues.

Table 8.1: Issues Related to Access to Information

> "Healthy aging and what is available for seniors. You can put all this information in the community centre. You can put it in the churches, but there are people who cannot get out of the building they are in."

Health Care

Participants expressed concern about recent federal and provincial decisions that are leading to a demise of the principles of Medicare. They were also concerned about reductions in federal transfers to provincial health plans. Participants related health issues to concerns about the state of long-term care and home care services. Coupled with these were concerns regarding the continued ability of seniors to access the health services they need and to make decisions about their own care and where they receive it. Access to required drugs was also a common concern.

In some localities, participants identified ageism among health care professionals and their perception of seniors as unable to understand their health care issues. In most localities, participants thought that there should be special training on seniors' issues for health care professionals. With the increasing demographic of older Canadians, the need for such training and education is apparent. Table 8.2 provides an illustrative statement by seniors.

Table 8.2: Issues Related to Health Care

> "So then you get cuts in services ... lying on gurneys in hospital hallways and having to wait for surgery and not getting adequate care because there are not enough backup staff, nurses, and technicians ... staff are overworked and can't give tender loving care."

Housing

Seniors were especially concerned about the lack of housing options for seniors. They tied housing to financial independence and autonomy, and the ability to access social and health services. Seniors need to be able to choose where and how they live, and not to have decisions forced upon them by others. Participants made numerous suggestions for increasing the housing stock. Underlying all of these actions was the political will to create more affordable housing for seniors and other Canadians. Table 8.3 provides an illustrative finding.

Table 8.3: Issues Related to Housing

"Canada should have a policy that everybody should know about, that this is what we stand for. We need to have a clear policy on what being a Canadian citizen means in terms of housing and any other issues ... Money from the surplus should reactivate a federal commitment to housing."

Income Security

Participants identified income security, particularly for senior women, as a serious issue. It represented the difference between independence and dependence on others, and most importantly the ability to remain in one's own home in the community. Women and immigrants may not have worked, or worked at jobs that did not provide pensions. Economic issues were seen largely in terms of pension plans and having enough money to remain active. They frequently considered existing pensions such as the Canada Pension Plan, Old Age Security, and the Guaranteed Annual Income as insufficient. Participants across localities recommended indexing these plans to inflation. Table 8.4 provides an illustrative finding.

Table 8.4: Issues Related to Income

"So once they are in [a retirement home] it gets to be expensive, and the funds run out. A lot of families say they don't have the heart to tell their mom and so somehow the burden falls onto the kids, and they are putting up extra money or paying for the rent."

Transportation

Transportation and the attendant issue of mobility are important issues for seniors. Participants linked these issues to avoiding loneliness and isolation, particularly among those suffering chronic health problems, recently widowed, or living alone. They identified good public transit as key to linking seniors to recreation activities and support networks. Participants considered public transit and volunteer drivers as means to help seniors with mobility difficulties to get around their cities to access services they need and participate in the life of their cities.

Barriers to Change

All locations identified ageism as a significant barrier. Many attributed this difficulty to prevailing attitudes towards seniors, particularly through the perpetuation of myths about seniors. Participants linked ageism to older adults' lack of political voice. Many argued that society does not value seniors for their wisdom from life experience. Participants called for recognition of seniors and appropriate representation of seniors in public consultations. Governments need to consult seniors and include them in decision-making processes, particularly on decisions that affect the well-being of seniors.

DISCUSSION

The seven cities involved in this research differ with respect to services offered, local political trends, and institutions. Each study used somewhat different questions and procedures. It is therefore striking how similar the findings are across locations. These findings suggest that the research approach applied is, first of all, robust in its power to detect important seniors' issues. The findings suggest common needs exist among seniors that are not being met by local authorities.

Seniors complained that governments do not listen to their voices. This finding is consistent with evidence of a diminishing role of civil society in public decision-making processes in western nations.[4,21] Increasingly, Canadian governments limit opportunities for civil society actors to influence legislation and public policy.

This is most apparent in the changing role of government in the areas of housing and health care that seniors identified as problematic. In both areas, provincial governments increasingly invite private sector involvement.[22,23] For example, the Ontario government opened long-term care community services to market competition. Service providers with a long history of non-profit service provision must now compete for contracts with private for-profit corporations.

CONCLUSIONS

The Seniors Quality of Life Project enabled seniors to identify and explore the determinants of their quality of life. The findings across localities and seniors' ability to report these findings demonstrate the usefulness of the determinants of health perspective and the participatory research methodological approach.[24]

Seniors can examine broad policy issues and identify how governments, service agencies, and communities can promote seniors' quality of life. These approaches provide rich areas for public health inquiry and action to improve the health and well-being of our growing older population.[25]

Appendix: Questions Asked in Three Seniors Quality of Life Studies

	Montreal
1.	What contributes to your well-being, so that you and those in your community have a good quality of life?
2.	What are the events or situations that have diminished quality of life for you or for people living in your community?
3.	What are the events or situations that have improved quality of life for you or for people living in your community?
4.	Are there any measures that could be taken by you, your friends, or the organizations in which you participate that could make your life more pleasant?
5.	Do governments have a role to play in your life? Could you provide examples?
	Toronto
1.	What policy decisions being made by governments are affecting seniors' quality of life?
2.	How do these decisions affect the quality of life of seniors?
3.	What factors are influencing governments to make these decisions?
4.	What responses to these decisions could be made?
	Vancouver
1.	What things affect your life for better or worse?
2.	Which ones of these could be influenced by governments (federal, provincial, municipal, or regional)?
3.	What suggestions do you have for resolving these issues?

REFERENCES

1. Health Canada. *Dare to Age Well!* Ottawa, ON: Division of Aging and Seniors, 2001.

2. Lilley S. *Policies for Aging Population: An International Perspective.* Halifax, NS: Population and Public Health Branch, Atlantic Region, Health Canada, 2002, November.

3. National Forum on Health. *Building on the Legacy: Volume 2, Adults and Seniors.* Ottawa, ON: National Forum on Health, 1998.

4. Bryant, T., Raphael, D., Brown, I., Wheeler, J., Herman, R., Houston, J., et al. Opening up the public policy analysis process to the public: participatory policy research and Canadian seniors' quality of life. *Can Rev Soc Pol* 2001;48:35–67.

5. Lilley, S., Campbell, J.M. *Shifting Sands: The Changing Shape of Atlantic Canada.* 1999. A report on economic and demographic trends in Atlantic Canada and their impacts on seniors. Population Public Health Branch Atlantic Region (PPHB Atlantic), Health Canada, 1999.

6. Ulysse, P-J, Lesemann, F. *Population Aging: An Overview of the Past Thirty Years: Review of the Literature.* Health Canada, Health Promotion and Programs Branch, Population Health Directorate, Division of Aging and Seniors, 1997.

7. Quality of Life Research Unit Website. *The Seniors Quality of Life Project.* Toronto, ON: Centre for Health Promotion, 2001.

8. Bryant, T., Raphael, D., Brown, I., Cogan, T., Dallaire, C., Laforest, S., et al. *A Nation for All Ages? A Participatory Study of Canadian Seniors' Quality of Life in Seven Municipalities.* Toronto, ON: York University Centre for Health Studies, 2002. Online at http://www.yorku.ca/ychs/seniorsfinalreport.pdf.

9. Health Canada. *The Population Health Template: Key Elements and Actions that Define a Population Health Approach.* Strategic Policy Directorate, Population and Public Health Branch, Health Canada, 2001. Online at http://www.hc-sc.gc.ca/hppb/phdd/pdf/discussion_paper.pdf.

10. Wilkinson, R., Marmot, M. *Social Determinants of Health: The Solid Facts*, 2nd edition. Copenhagen, Denmark: World Health Organization (WHO), Europe Office, 2003. Online at http://www.who.dk/document/e81384.pdf.

11. Marmot, M., Wilkinson, R. *Social Determinants of Health.* Oxford, UK: Oxford University Press, 2000.

12. Minkler, M., Wallerstein, N., Hall, B. *Community Based Participatory Research for Health.* San Francisco, CA: Jossey-Bass, 2002.

13. Lindstrom, B. Quality of life: A model for evaluating "Health for All." *Soz Praventivmed* 1992;37:301–6.

14. Raphael, D., Brown, I., Renwick, R., Rootman, I. Quality of life: what are the implications for health promotion? *Am J Health Behav* 1997;21(2):118–28.

15. Canadian Policy Research Networks. *Asking Citizens what Matters for Quality of Life in Canada: A Rural Lens*. Ottawa, ON: Canadian Policy Research Networks (CPRN), 2001 November. Online at http://www.cprn.com/en/theme-docs.cfm?theme=4.

16. Navarro, V., Shi, L. The political context of social inequalities and health. In: Navarro V (Ed.), *The Political Economy of Social Inequalities: Consequences for Health and Quality of Life*. Amityville, NY: Baywood, 2002.

17. Federation of Canadian Municipalities. *Quality of Life Reporting System: Quality of Life in Canadian Communities*. Federation of Canadian Municipalities (FCM), 1999. Online at http://www.fcm.ca/english/communications/qualitylife.htm.

18. Michalski, J.H. *Asking Citizens what Matters for Quality of Life in Canada: Results of CPRN's Public Dialogue Process*. Ottawa, ON: Canadian Policy Research Networks (CPRN), 2001. Online at http://www.cprn.com/en/doc.cfm?doc=48.

19. Health Canada. *Taking Action on Population Health: A Position Paper for Health Promotion and Programs Branch Staff*. Ottawa, ON: Health Canada, 1998. Online at http://www.hc-sc.gc.ca/hppb/phdd/pdf/tad_e.pdf.

20. Lincoln, Y.S., Cuba, E.G. *Naturalistic Inquiry*. Beverly Hills, CA: Sage Publications, 1985.

21. Bryant, T. Role of knowledge in public health and health promotion policy change. *Health Prom Int* 2002; 17(1):89–98.

22. Armstrong, P., Amaratunga, C., Bernier, J., Grant, K., Pederson, A., Wilson, K. *Exposing Privatization: Women and Health Care Reform in Canada*. Toronto, ON: Garamond, 2002.

23. Bryant, T. The current state of housing as a social determinant of health. *Policy Options* 2003; March:52–56.

24. Raphael, D. (Ed). *Social Determinants of Health: Canadian Perspectives*. Toronto, ON: Canadian Scholars Press Inc., 2004.

25. Lessard, R. *Prevent, Cure, Care—Challenges of an Ageing Society. 1999 Annual Report on the Health of the Montreal Population*. Montreal, QC: Direction de la santé publique de Montréal-Centre, 1999. Online at http://www.santepub-mtl.qc.ca/Publication/rapportannuel/1999/intro1999eng.pdf.

CHAPTER 9

The Welfare State as a Determinant of Women's Health

Dennis Raphael and Toba Bryant

OVERVIEW

Quality of life is a holistic construct that views human health and well-being within the contexts of proximal and distal environments [1]. It combines elements of broad societal indicators with the actual lived experience of people [2]. Emphasis is increasingly being placed on considering quality of life in particular relation to national and local policy environments [3].

Davies et al. [4] consider how women's economic vulnerability in nations such as Canada makes them especially sensitive to regressive changes in social policy [5]. Women in their assigned role of caregivers of both their children and relatives are most likely to be impacted by changes in social assistance policies, changes to employment insurance eligibility, and provision of health and social services, among others [6]. These are the kinds of policies that show systematic differences among nations with social welfare versus market orientations to social policy.

While a wide range of conceptualisations of quality of life are available, the *Canadian Policy Research Networks* recently identified—based on a broad consensus-building exercise—priority themes for considering quality of life [7]. These themes are—in order of identified importance—political rights and general values, health, including health care, education, environment, social programs, personal well-being, community, economy and employment, and government. These themes show many similarities with the increasingly important literature on the social determinants of health. A social determinants of health perspective is increasingly being applied to national approaches to the formulation of health policy [8,9]. This is especially the case in the Scandinavian nations.

In this paper, we consider the extent to which these quality of life issues are supported by governmental action in Canada and four comparison nations. The information relevant to these issues comes primarily from two types of data sources: indicator analyses from international reports and intensive and detailed policy analyses of a policy issue of particular importance to women: childcare provision.

Canadian data are contrasted with those from Denmark, Sweden, the UK, and the US. These nations have been chosen for an obvious reason: Denmark and Sweden are nations with a predominantly social welfare approach to social policy, especially in relation to issues of concern to women; the UK and US have a predominantly market-oriented approach to these same issues [10]. The case is argued that nations with a predominantly welfare state orientation are more likely to support the quality of life themes relevant to women's health and well-being.

Political Rights and General Values

The quality of political rights and general values is not easily captured in indicator analyses. In a recent work, we considered these issues in relation to Canada's adherence to the *Convention to Eliminate All Forms of Discrimination Against Women* (CEDAW) [11,12]. The conclusion reached in various reports to the United Nations by Canadian women's groups and most recently by the United Nations CEDAW Committee itself is that Canada is not working to implement the provisions of the Convention through the exercise of women's political rights:

> The Committee acknowledges the State party's complex federal, provincial and territorial political and legal struc-
> tures. However, it underlines the federal Government's principal responsibility in implementing the Convention. The Committee is concerned that the federal Government does not seem to have the power to ensure that governments establish legal and other measures in order to fully

implement the Convention in a coherent and consistent manner ([13], p. 5).

This UN report is consistent with a number of reports produced by women's groups in Canada that speak of the systematic denial of women's political and economic rights resulting from government actions [14–18]. Similar official and shadow CEDAW reports are available for Sweden and the UK [19–21]. The US is the only industrialised country that has not ratified CEDAW.

Health, Including Health Care

A number of indicators from the United Nations' *Human Development Report (HDR)* [22] map onto this quality of life theme. The overall *Human Development Index* takes into account general life expectancy, GDP per capita, and education. Table 9.1 shows that Canada performs very well in the overall index, though it has lost its #1 rank of the last few years. However, a more sensitive indicator—*human and income poverty*—which considers the incidence of poverty and numbers of citizens lacking functional literacy, finds Canada occupying a position midway between the social welfare nations of Denmark and Sweden and the market-oriented UK and US. This pattern repeats itself in many of the analyses that follow.

The *HDR* also provides a number of indicators of national commitment to health. As compared to the social welfare nations, Canada has fewer physicians and spends less public money on health care. However, with the relatively high percentage of funds being expended privately, Canada spends more on health care than all nations except the US.

Education

As noted in Table 9.1, Canada scores high on a relative index of enrolment density, yet falls behind the social welfare nations on an indicator of functional literacy. Table 9.2 shows the *HDR* indicators for public spending on education. Canada scores midway between the social welfare and market economy nations.

Table 9.1: Human Development and Human and Income Poverty and Commitment to Health in Canada and Four Comparison Nations, 1999

	Canada	Denmark	Sweden	UK	US
HDI (rank)	3	14	2	13	6
Life expectancy	78.8	76.2	79.7	77.7	77.0
GDP per capita	27840	27627	24277	23509	34142
Education index	0.98	0.98	0.99	0.99	0.98
Human poverty index (rank)	12	5	1	15	17
Percentage in poverty (%)	12.3	9.5	6.7	15.1	15.8
<50% median income (%)	12.8	9.2	6.6	13.4	16.9
<Functional literacy (%)	16.6	9.6	7.5	21.8	20.7
Adequate sanitation (%)	100	100	100	100	100
Physicians/100,000	229	290	311	164	279
Public Can$ as percentage of GDP (%)	6.6	6.9	6.6	5.8	5.7
Private Can$ as percentage of GDP (%)	2.7	1.5	1.3	1.2	7.1
Total Can$ as percentage of GDP (%)	9,3	8.4	7.9	7.0	12.8
Spending per capita	1939	2785	2145	1675	4271

Source: HDR [22].

Table 9.2: Commitment to Education: Public Spending on Education in Canada and Four Comparison Nations, 1995–1997

	Canada	Denmark	Sweden	UK	US
Public education (% GDP)	6.9	8.1	8.3	5.3	5.4
Spending as percentage total government	12.9	13.1	12.2	11.6	14.4

Source: HDR [22].

Environment

The *HDR* provides two environmental indicators. As shown in Table 9.3, Canada is the highest national per capita consumer of electricity and second only to the US in per capita carbon dioxide emissions.

Table 9.3: Energy and the Environment Indicators in Canada and Four
Comparison Nations, 1997

	Canada	Denmark	Sweden	UK	US
Electricity consumption	15260	6030	14138	5384	11994
Carbon dioxide emissions in tons per capita	15.3	10.1	5.5	9.2	19.9

Source: HDR [22].

Social Programs

A wide number of indicators are available related to national commitment to social programs. Women's well-being is especially influenced
by the presence of social programs due to their greater economic
vulnerability and multiple roles. Table 9.4 provides data related to
public spending on broad social policy areas and provides the value
of unemployment assistance benefits for short-term (one month) and
longer-term recipients. Later sections examine issues of childcare in
greater detail. Outside of the US, Canada provides less net replacement value for short- and long-term assistance recipients than all
other comparison nations.

Personal Well-being

National statistics from surveys on incidence of crime are available
and are presented in Table 9.5. No clear pattern is seen among the
nations in these statistics.

Income distribution is increasingly being identified as an indicator of societal and personal well-being [24–27]. A number of
indicators are related to income distribution and incidence of
poverty among nations and among populations within Canada
(Table 9.6).

While Canada is second only to the US in GDP per capita, its
distribution of income is midway between the social welfare and
market-oriented nations. The Gini index ranges from 0.00 (perfect
equality) to 1.00 (all income controlled by one person). It usually is

multiplied by 100 to give a range from 0 to 100. Table 9.7 provides insight into the situation of single women in Canada, though these figures do not make a distinction between male and female single parents.

Table 9.4: Public Social Expenditure by Broad Social Policy Areas as Percentage of GDP, 1997, and Net Replacement Rates at the Earnings Levels of Two-thirds of an Average Production Worker in the First Month of Benefit Receipt and for Long-term Benefit Recipients in Canada and Four Comparison Nations, 1999

	Canada	Denmark	Sweden	UK	US
Public social expenditure					
Cash benefits (%)	10.2	16.8	18.2	13.6	9.0
Services (%)	6.7	13.7	15.1	8.0	7.0
Total spending (%)	16.9	30.5	33.3	21.6	16.0
Net replacement earnings for unemployed					
Single person					
Short-term (%)	62	89	77	73	59
Long-term (%)	35	67	84	73	10
Married couple					
Short-term (%)	65	94	77	88	59
Long-term (%)	57	94	100	88	18
Couple—two children					
Short-term (%)	69	95	90	83	51
Long-term (%)	77	92	100	95	61
Lone parent—two children					
Short-term (%)	67	89	96	69	51
Long-term (%)	77	82	100	81	51

Cash benefits include pensions and income supports to the working age population. Services include health and other social services. Source: SGR [23].

A detailed analysis of the current state of Canadian women in re-gards to economic well-being is provided in a report by Hadley [28]. In 1997, 56% of all female lone parents had incomes below Statistics Canada low-income cut-offs—an indicator similar to the poverty marker used by the Organisation for Economic Co-operation and Development (OECD).

Table 9.5: Reports of Being a Victim of Crime as Percentage of Total Population in Canada and Four Comparison Nations, 1999

	Canada	Denmark	Sweden	UK	US
Property crime (%)	10.4	7.6	8.4	12.2	10.0
Robbery (%)	0.9	0.7	0.9	1.2	0.6
Sexual assault (females) (%)	0.8	0.4	1.1	0.9	0.4
Assault (%)	2.3	1.4	1.2	2.8	1.2
Total crime (%)	23.8	23.0	24.7	26.4	21.1

Source: HDR [22].

Table 9.6: Income and Income Distribution in Canada and Four Comparison Nations, 1999

	Canada	Denmark	Sweden	UK	US
GDP per capita	27840	27627	24277	23509	34142
Income share— poorest 10%	2.8%	3.6%	3.7%	2.6%	1.8%
Income share— poorest 20%	7.5%	9.6%	9.6%	6.6%	5.2%
Income share— richest 10%	23.8%	20.5%	20.1%	20.5%	30.5%
Income share— richest 20%	39.3%	34.5%	34.5%	43.0%	46.4%
Richest 10% to poorest 10%	8.5%	5.7%	5.4%	10.4%	16.6%
Richest 20% to poorest 20%	5.2%	3.6%	3.6%	6.5%	9.0%
Gini index	31.5%	24.7%	25.0%	36.1%	40.8%

Source: HDR [22].

Table 9.7: Percentage of Persons Living in Parental Households with Income Below 50% of Median Adjustable Income of the Entire Population (Poverty Rates) in Canada and Four Comparison Nations, 1994

	Canada	Denmark	Sweden	UK	US
Single parents working (%)	63	74	87	47	73
Poverty rates					
Non-working single (%)	72	34	24	65	73
Working single (%)	26	10	4	23	39

Source: SGR [23].

Economy and Employment

As noted, Canadian per capital income is second to the US among the comparison nations. However, income is distributed more unequally than in the social welfare nations. The following tables provide evidence concerning income inequality between men and women and level of unemployment in Canada and the comparison nations.

Canadian women, like women elsewhere, do not participate in paid employment activity to a similar extent as men. Yet they spend more hours overall on combined employment and household duties than men [29]. Canadian unemployment rates—applying to those able and/ or seeking employment—are high as compared to both the social welfare and market economy-oriented nations (Table 9.8). The female rate is similar to that of men. Youth unemployment rates are also relatively high in Canada, though the female rate is lower than that for males. Finally, Canada's percentage of unemployed that are long-term unemployed—this group does not include those with disabilities—is relatively low as compared to all nations except the US. The low US rate may reflect the lack of available benefits for the long-term unemployed that may either force individuals to find employment of some sort or make such long-term unemployed individuals "invisible."

Table 9.8: Gender Inequality in Economic Activity and Unemployment Levels in Canada and Four Comparison Nations, 1999

	Canada	Denmark	Sweden	UK	US
Female economic activity (%)	60.1	61.7	62.5	52.8	58.8
As percentage male rate (%)	82	84	89	74	81
Unemployment rate (%)	6.8	4.7	4.7	5.5	4.0
Female rate as percentage male rate (%)	96	123	87	79	105
Youth unemployment (%)	12.6	6.7	11.9	11.8	9.3
Female rate as percentage male rate (%)	81	107	93	77	92
Long-term as percentage total rate (%)					
Male	12.2	20.1	33.1	33.7	6.7
Female	10.0	20.0	27.7	19.0	5.3

Source: HDR [22].

Table 9.9 provides figures related to spending in support of government action to support prospects of gainful employment, job skills of the labour force, and the functioning of the labour force. These include public employment services and administration, labour-market training, youth measures, subsidized employment, and measures for the disabled. Canada is very low in comparison to the social welfare nations.

Table 9.9: Active and Passive Labour-market Public Spending as Percentage of GDP, Canada and Four Comparison Nations, 1999

	Canada	Denmark	Sweden	UK	US
Active spending (%)	0.50	1.75	1.8	0.4	0.2
Passive spending (%)	1.0	3.1	1.7	0.75	0.25
Total spending (%)	1.5	4.85	3.5	1.15	0.45

Source: SGR [23].

Within Canada, an analysis has provided insights into the income gap between men and women [28]. In 1998, 30% of men in Canada had earned income less than $13,786(CAD). The corresponding figure for women was 50%. Similarly in 1998, 29% of men had earned income over $32,367(CAD); the figure for women was 11%. Interestingly, whether one worked in a unionized job significantly influenced income level. Among women who worked in full-time unionized positions only 1.5% had income less than $13,786(CAD). The corresponding figure for full-time women workers in non-unionized jobs was 14%. The wage gap between men and women in full-time unionized jobs was 18%; in non-unionized full-time jobs, 25%. These data are consistent with the analysis of Baker and Fortin [30] concerning the enhancing effects for income enjoyed by women in unionized positions.

In the *Society at a Glance Report (SGR)*, the OECD calculated the gender wage gap for member nations from the mid- to late-1990s in terms of female median full-time earnings as a percentage of male median full-time earnings. The differences were as follows: Canada, 30%; Denmark, 12%; Sweden, 17%; the UK, 23%; and the US, 22%.

Finally, Hadley considered various indicators of income inequality between Canadian men and women. Women's income as a percentage of men's income for full-time, full-year employment was 72.5%; for hourly wages, 80%; for those with university degrees, 74%; for all men and women, 63%; and median after tax income, 61%.

Government

The United Nations provides a gender empowerment index and provides data on women's participation in government. These data are provided in Table 9.10.

Canada ranks relatively high in this index. Nonetheless, Canada's seats in parliaments held by women is low, though Canada does comparatively well on the other ratings. A consistent picture emerges from these analyses. Canada performs well in just about every indicator of general quality of life and women's quality of life as compared to the UK and the US. Canada does not perform well in relation to the values on a number of indicators of Denmark and Sweden. The next section continues this examination of national policy differences in relation to a key issue relevant to women's quality of life: childcare.

Table 9.10: Gender Empowerment in Canada and Four Comparison Nations, 2001

	Canada	Denmark	Sweden	UK	US
Overall rank	7	4	3	16	11
Seats in parliament (%)	23.6	37.4	42.7	17.0	13.8
Female legislators, senior officials, managers (%)	35	23	29	33	45
Female professional and technical workers (%)	53	50	49	45	53
Ratio female:male income	0.62	0.70	0.68	0.61	0.62
Women at ministerial level (%)	24.3	45.0	55.0	33.3	31.8
Lower house (%)	20.6	37.4	42.7	18.4	14.0
Upper house (%)	32.4	15.6	N/A	15.6	13.0

Source: HDR [22].

CHILDCARE: EXAMINING THE FACTORS SUPPORTING WOMEN'S QUALITY OF LIFE

Childcare is consistently identified as a key concern of Canadian women [31]. It appears that the policy approaches governments take towards childcare mirror their general approach towards women's health, well-being, and quality of life.

At the end of the 1990's there has been a convergence of ideas about why and how early childhood care and education are important not only for individual Canadian children and families but for Canadian society at large ... There is broad recognition that a strategy for developing early childhood services that offer *both* early childhood education to strengthen healthy development for children *and* childcare to support mothers' labour force participation is in the public interest ([32], preface, emphasis in original).

The data and analysis related to the availability and quality of childcare for Canadian women and those from the four comparisons nations come from two primary sources. These are the *Early Childhood Care and Education in Canada: Provinces and Territories 1998* report produced by the Childcare Resource and Research Unit at the University of Toronto [32] and outputs from the OECD *Thematic Review of Early Childhood Education and Care Policy* [33]. The latter was a 12-nation study of OECD nations that did not include Canada. Data from these reports were combined to provide a composite picture of the nature of childcare in Canada and the comparison nations.

Women, Motherhood, and Employment in Canada and Elsewhere

Besides the obvious human development benefits of providing children with stimulating, safe, and quality childcare, the availability of childcare allows women to have gainful employment. Table 9.11 shows the percentage of married/cohabiting mothers and percentage of lone mothers that are employed in Canada and the four comparison nations, while Table 9.12 summarizes paid maternity leave benefits. Table 9.13 shows percentage of children receiving out-of-home childcare.

Table 9.11: Percentage of Canadian and Other Nation Mothers Employed as Function of Habitation Status, 1996

	Canada[a]	Denmark	Sweden	UK	US
Married/cohabiting (%)	71	84	80	62	68
Lone mothers (%)	63	69	70	41	66

Source: [33]. [a]Canadian figures for 2000 from Statistics Canada (Statistics Canada, 2002).

Table 9.12: Provisions for Paid Maternity Leave in Canada and Four Comparison Nations, 1995–1996

Canada	Fifteen weeks paid at 55%. In 2001, eligibility for benefits was increased by the Federal government to 52 weeks.
Denmark	Twenty-eight weeks paid at 100% salary.
Sweden	Fifty-two weeks paid at 80% salary.
UK	Twelve weeks paid at 90%.
US	Unpaid.

Source: [34–43].

Table 9.13: Proportion of Young Children who Use Out-of-home Childcare Facilities up to Mandatory Schooling Age in Canada and Four Comparison Nations, 1998 and 1999

	Canada	Denmark	Sweden	UK	US
0–3 year olds (%)	44	58	48	2	26
3 years to mandatory age (%)	50	83	79	60	71

Source: [44].

CHILDCARE AND EARLY CHILD EDUCATION POLICY SITUATION

About half of Canadian children are in out-of-home childcare arrangements; significantly less than that seen for Denmark and Sweden with its state-supportive system. The figures for the UK are strikingly low. Bertram and Pascal [45] note that "Current provision of education and care for under 3s in the UK is uneven, of mixed quality and in short supply ... These issues are recognised by the Government's National Childcare Strategy which aims to encourage growth of quality provision for under 3s" (p. 26).

Canada: Canadian governments provide universal education for children ages 5–6, but for those under 5 years of age, government-supported childcare may be available for those with special needs, poor, or working parents. The funding strategies are mixed, but come primarily from parent fees. Only 10% of Canadian children have access to regulated childcare [44].

According to the International Reform Monitor [34–43], Canadian provincial governments provided subsidised childcare for some low-income parents, but supply is inadequate to the demand and cut-backs have worsened the situation in some provinces. Most families still must use private, unregulated childcare. The most enlightened province is Quebec, where subsidised childcare has been introduced for all children. The pursuit of family-friendly workplaces on the part of employers remains in its infancy in Canada. The National Child Benefit is available to low-income families but most provinces claw these back from families on social assistance.

Denmark: Danish governments provide universal education for children 5-7, and provide childcare from 6 months to 6 years for working parents. Government funding is supplemented by income-related parent fees to a maximum of 20-30% of costs. Denmark provides comprehensive provision of social services to support families. There are day nurseries, municipal day care centres, kindergartens, youth recreation centres, and age-integrated institutions. Extra benefits are provided for single-parent families.

Sweden: Swedish governments provide universal childcare and early childhood education for children from birth to 6 years of age. Funding is provided by federal and local governments. Sweden provides a very good infrastructure of support services to working parents. There is a parental allowance of 60 days per year per child for sick children under 12 years of age. Fees for childcare expenses are being lowered and unemployed parents are guaranteed three hours of childcare per day. Extra benefits are provided for single-parent families.

UK: The UK provides universal education for children 3-4 years of age. From ages 0 to 4, childcare outside of school is available only for special needs and poor families with funding coming from governments or income-related fees. The UK is implementing new measures to assist employed single parents, such as a child tax credit to obtain childcare.

US: The US provides free education for children aged 5. For children from 0 to 4 years of age, childcare is available for special needs, poor, welfare, and working parents. Funding comes from governments but parent fees cover 76% of costs. Many parents in the US are unable to afford such care [46]. Some US employers offer subsidized childcare facilities; the vast majority do not. After welfare reform, more low-income families with children need to find and hold jobs. Federal employees are entitled to 24 hour work-leave for child-related activities.

CONCLUSION: THE WELFARE STATE AND WOMEN'S QUALITY OF LIFE

The findings concerning women's quality of life in Canada are consistent with the analysis of Fast and Keating [47] who identified four key changes in the Canadian policy environment: Reduced government expenditure on health, income security, and social services; push towards the privatization of health and continuing care; shift from institutional to community-based health and community care; and increased geographic inequity in health and social service delivery.

It is obvious from our analysis that policies associated with the social welfare states of Denmark and Sweden are clearly beneficial to women and enhance their quality of life. Yet, in Canada there is increasing evidence of a shift in policy orientation towards the market-oriented policies associated with the UK and the US [48]. Such a direction does not bode well for Canadian women and their quality of life [49]. Caregiving in the US is seen to be in a crisis situation and has strong implications for the quality of American women's and their children's lives [50,51].

The Canadian Policy Research Network's quality of life initiative identified cross-cutting themes of accessibility; personal security/control; availability; and equity/fairness. Women's quality of life is influenced by the extent to which women have access to the resources that are normally available to those within a society [52]. The roles that society thrusts upon Canadian women of child rearing and caregiving makes access to these resources—such as childcare and home care—especially important [53]. Equality of opportunity is an empty phrase unless society—and the governments it elects—is willing to make the policy decisions that support women in their lives [54]. This is the meaning of equity and fairness.

In terms of contemporary analyses of women's quality of life, these policy changes in Canada—and elsewhere—have been considered for their impact on Canadian women's quality of life [55–57]. These kinds of policy-oriented quality of life analyses are rarely done in relation to women's health [58–60]. As such, these analyses should complement more traditional approaches to considering women's health and well-being in Canada and other nations [61].

REFERENCES

1. Lindstrom, B. Quality of life: A model for evaluating health for all. Soz Praventivmed 1992;37:301–6.

2. Raphael, D., Renwick, R., Brown, I., Steinmetz, B., Sehdev, H., Phillips, S. Making the links between community structure and individual well-being. Community quality of life in Riverdale, Toronto, Canada. Health and Place 2001;7(3): 17–34.

3. Navarro, V., editor. The political economy of social inequalities: Consequences for health and quality of life. Amityville (NY): Baywood; 2002.

4. Davies, L., McMullin, J.A., Avison, W.R., Cassidy, G.L. Social policy, gender inequality and poverty. Ottawa: Status of Women Canada; 2001.

5. Day, S. Brodsky, G. Women and the equality deficit: The impact of restructuring Canada's social programs. Ottawa: Status of Women Canada; 1998.

6. Côté, D. Who will be responsible for providing care? The impact of the shift to ambulatory care and of social economy policies on Quebec women. Ottawa: Status of Women Canada; 1998.

7. Michalski, J.H. Asking citizens what matters for quality of life in Canada: Results of CPRN's public dialogue process. Ottawa: Canadian Policy Research Networks; 2001.

8. Raphael, D. Addressing the social determinants of health in Canada: Bridging the gap between research findings and public policy. Policy Options 2003;24(3):35–40.

9. Raphael, D., editor. Social determinants of health: Canadian perspectives. Toronto: Canadian Scholars Press; 2004.

10. Navarro, V., Shi, L. The political context of social inequalities and health. Social Science and Medicine 2001; 52:481–91.

11. United Nations. In: Proceedings of the Convention on the Elimination of all Forms of Discrimination Against Women (1979). New York: United Nations.

12. Raphael, D., Bryant, T. The quality of women's life in Canada. Toronto: York Centre for Health Studies; 2003.

13. United Nations Committee on the Elimination of Discrimination Against Women. Concluding Remarks on the Canada Report. Twenty-Eighth Session, 13–31 January 2003.

14. Canadian Advisory Committee on the Status of Women (1977). Parallel Report to the Second Report of Canada to the United Nations Committee on the Elimination of all Forms of Discrimination Against Women. Ottawa: Canadian Advisory Committee on the Status of Women.

15. McPhedran, M., Bazilli, S., Erickson, M., Byrnes, A. The first CEDAW impact study. Toronto: York University Centre for Feminist Studies; 2000.

16. National Action Committee on the Status of Women (1990). Parallel Report to the Second Report of Canada to the UN Committee on the Elimination of all Forms of Discrimination Against Women. Ottawa: National Action Committee on the Status of Women.

17. Stienstraq, D., Roberts, B. Little but lip service: assessing Canada's implementation of its international obligations for women's equality. Ottawa: Canadian Advisory Committee on the Status of Women; 1993.

18. Waldorf, L., Bazilli, S. The CEDAW impact study: Canada. Toronto: York University Centre for Feminist Studies; 2003. Retrieved 1 September 2003, from the World Wide Web: http://www.iwrp.org/CEDAW_Impact_Study.htm.

19. United Nations Division for Advancement of Women (2003). CEDAW Convention National Reports. New York: National Division for Advancement of Women. Retrieved 1 September 2003, from the World Wide Web: http://www.un.org/womenwatch/daw/cedaw/reports.htm.

20. Swedish Foundation for Human Rights (2002). Alternative report to the expert committee with respect to Sweden's commitments under the international covenant on economic, social and cultural rights. Stockholm: Swedish Foundation for Human Rights. Retrieved 1 September 2003, from the World Wide Web: http://www.humanrights.se/svenska/ESK-rapp.pdf.

21. Women's Resource Centre (2002). Women's Resource Centre Response to the Women's National Commission on the Government's Draft 5th CEDAW Report to the United Nations. London: Women's Resource Center. Retrieved 1 September 2003, from the World Wide Web: http://www.wrc.org.uk/Word&rtfs/WRC%20Response%20to%20Shadow%20Report%20Dec%20%2002.rtf.

22. United Nations Development Program (2002). Human Development Report 2002. Geneva: United Nations Development Program.

23. Organization for Economic Co-operation and Development (2001). Society at a glance: OECD social indicators 2001 edition. Paris: Organization for Economic Co-operation and Development.

24. Evans, R.G., Barer, M., Marmor, T.R. Why are some people healthy and others not? The determinants of health of populations. New York: Aldine de Gruyter; 1994.

25. Raphael, D. Health effects of economic inequality. Canadian Review of Social Policy 1999;44:25–40.

26. Raphael, D. Health inequalities in Canada: Current discourses and implications for public health action. Critical Public Health 2000;10:193–216.

27. Wilkinson, R.G. Unhealthy societies: The afflictions of inequality. New York: Routledge; 1996.

28. Hadley, K. And we still ain't satisfied: A status report for 2001. Gender inequality in Canada. Toronto: Centre for Social Justice; 2001.

29. Clark, W. Economic Gender Equality Indicators 2000. Ottawa: Canadian Social Trends; 2001.

30. Baker, M., Fortin, N. Gender composition and wages: Why is Canada different from the United States? Working Papers. Toronto: Department of Economics, University of Toronto; 1998.

31. Tyyska, V. Women, citizenship and Canadian childcare policy in the 1990s. Occasional paper 13. Childcare Resource and Research Unit. Toronto: University of Toronto Childcare Resource and Research Unit; 2001.

32. Friendly, M. Early childhood care and education in Canada, 1998. Childcare Resource and Research Unit, University of Toronto; 2000.

33. Neuman, M. Early childhood education and care policy: international trends and developments [special issue]. International Journal of Educational Research 2000;33(1).

34. International Reform Monitor. Social policy, labour market policy and industrial relations, long-term care: Canada. Bertelsmann Foundation; 2002.

35. International Reform Monitor. Social policy, labour market policy and industrial relations, long-term care: Denmark. Bertelsmann Foundation; 2002.

36. International Reform Monitor. Social policy, labour market policy and industrial relations, long-term care: Sweden. Bertelsmann Foundation; 2002.

37. International Reform Monitor. Social policy, labour market policy and industrial relations, long-term care: United Kingdom. Bertelsmann Foundation; 2002.

38. International Reform Monitor. Social policy, labour market policy and industrial relations, long-term care: United States. Bertelsmann Foundation; 2002.

39. International Reform Monitor. Social policy, labour market policy and industrial relations, family policy: Canada. Bertelsmann Foundation; 2002.

40. International Reform Monitor. Social policy, labour market policy and industrial relations, family policy: Denmark. Bertelsmann Foundation.

41. International Reform Monitor. Social policy, labour market policy and industrial relations, family policy: Sweden. Bertelsmann Foundation; 2002.

42. International Reform Monitor. Social policy, labour market policy and industrial relations, family policy: United Kingdom. Bertelsmann Foundation; 2002.

43. International Reform Monitor. Social policy, labour market policy and industrial relations, family policy: United States. Bertelsmann Foundation; 2002.

44. Kamerman, S. Early childhood education and care: an overview of developments in the OECD countries. International Journal of Educational Research 2000;33:7–29.

45. Bertram, T., Pascal, C. The OECD thematic review of early childhood education and care: background report for the United Kingdom. Paris: Organization for Economic Co-operation and Development; 2000.

46. Shulman, K. Issue brief: The high cost of childcare puts quality care out of reach for many families. Washington (DC): Children's Defense Fund; 2000.

47. Fast, J.E., Keating, N.C. Family caregiving and consequences for carers: towards a policy research agenda. CPRN Discussion Paper No. F10. Ottawa: Canadian Policy Research Networks; 2000.

48. Bryant, T., Raphael, D., Brown, I., Wheeler, J., Herman, R., Houston, J., et al. Opening up the public policy analysis process to the public: Participatory policy research and Canadian seniors' quality of life. Canadian Review of Social Policy 2001;48:35–57.

49. Townson, M. A report card on women and poverty. Ottawa: Canadian Centre for Policy Alternatives; 2002.

50. Heywood, J. The widening gap: Why America's working families are in jeopardy and what can be done about it. New York: Basic Books; 2000.

51. Heywood, J. Caregiving in Crisis. Boston Review 2002;27(1):4–13.

52. Raphael, D., Brown, I., Renwick, R., Rootman, I., Quality of life: What are the implications for health promotion? American Journal of Health Behavior 1997;21:118–28.

53. International Labour Organization. Maternity Protection at Work: Revision of the Maternity Protection Convention (Revised), 1952 (No. 103), and Recommendation, 1952 (No. 95) Report V (1). Geneva: International Labour Office.

54. Jones, E. Rothney, A. Women's health and social inequality. Ottawa: Canadian Centre for Policy Alternatives; 2001.

55. Bashevkin, S. Women on the defensive: Living through conservative times. Chicago: University of Chicago Press; 1998.

56. Bashevkin, S. Welfare hot buttons: Women, work, and social policy reform. Toronto: University of Toronto Press; 2002.

57. National Council of Welfare. The cost of poverty. Ottawa: National Council of Welfare.

58. Donner, L. Women, income and health in Manitoba: An overview and ideas for action. Winnipeg: Women's Health Clinic; 2002.

59. Pederson, A. What makes us healthy, what makes us sick? Research Bulletin of the Centres of Excellence for Women's Health 2001;1(2):1 and 3.

60. Walter, V. Lenton R, Mckeary M. Women's health in the context of women's lives. Ottawa: Health Canada; 1995.

61. Breitenbach, E. Research on women's health in Scotland: An overview. Edinburgh: Scottish Office Central Research Unit; 1999.

RECOMMENDED READINGS

1. Bryant, T., Raphael, D., Brown, I., Cogan, T., Dallaire, C., Laforest, S., McGowan, P., Richard, L., Thompson, L., & Young, J. (2002). *A nation for all ages? A participatory study of Canadian seniors' quality of life in seven municipalities.* Toronto: York Centre for Health Studies, York University. Available at www. utoronto.ca/seniors/seniorsfinalreport.pdf.

   This national project was funded by the Population Healthy Fund and provides a framework by which seniors can learn about the determinants of health and identify their effects upon their health and the health of those around them. The activities use a methodology that attempts to see the world through the eyes of seniors themselves. The report summarizes findings from seven Canadian cities and identifies common themes and their public policy implications

2. Federation of Canadian Municipalities. (1999). *The FCM quality of life reporting system: Quality of life in Canadian communities.* Ottawa: Federation of Canadian Municipalities. Available at http://www.fcm.ca//CMFiles/qol19991VSO-3272008-6325.pdf

   This report outlines the justification and key indicators for the quality of life reporting system. The purpose of the project is to provide evidence of important trends taking place across the municipal sector. By doing so the Quality of Life Reporting System (QOLRS) will ensure that municipal government is a strong partner in formulating public policy in Canada. The indicator domains are demographic and background information; affordable, appropriate housing; civic engagement; community and social infrastructure; education; employment; local economy; natural environment; personal and community health; personal financial security; and personal safety.

3. Federation of Canadian Municipalities (2004). *Highlights report.* Ottawa: Federation of Canadian Municipalities.

   The *Highlights Report* presents selected indicators from the QOLRS to show key changes from 1991 to 2001. The analysis found that quality of life in the 20 QOLRS member communities was at risk and had deteriorated for a significant number of people. The report portrays a rollercoaster period of severe economic decline between 1991 and 1996, followed by a general recovery in levels of income, falling poverty rates, and reduced housing affordability problems between 1996 and 2001.

4. Federation of Canadian Municipalities. (2004). *Quality of life in Canadian communities: Incomes, shelter and necessities.* Ottawa: Federation of Canadian Municipalities. Available at http://www.fcm.ca//CMFiles/nov1720041VJU-3272008-2356.pdf.

   This report focuses on a set of trends occurring between 1991 and 2001 related to personal incomes, shelter, and the affordability of basic needs. The report provides an in-depth analysis of the demographic groups more vulnerable to the effects of falling incomes, high rates of poverty, and more severe housing affordability challenges. A series of statistical charts and local stories from QOLRS member communities illustrate these broader trends.

5. Federation of Canadian Municipalities (2008). *Quality of life in Canadian communities: Trends and issues in affordable housing and homelessness.* Ottawa: Federation of Canadian Municipalities. Available at www.fcm.ca//CMFiles/qol20081VVM-3272008-3162.pdf.

   This reports focuses on trends related to housing and homelessness in 22 large and medium-sized municipalities and urban regions in Canada. Trend data are provided for the period 2000–2006, with some reference to trends dating back to 1991. A series of statistical charts and local stories from QOLRS member communities illustrate these trends.

6. Michalski, J. H. (2001). *Asking citizens what matters for quality of life in Canada: Results of CPRN's public dialogue process.* Ottawa: Canadian Policy Research Networks.

   This report summarizes the main components of the dialogue results, including a detailed thematic analysis of the content of the dialogue groups' discussions and an analysis of responses to questionnaires completed by participants both before and after the dialogue groups. It includes a summary of participants' general views about what constitutes quality of life in Canada, priority issue areas related to quality of life, appropriate indicators for measuring quality of life, and satisfaction with quality of life issues.

7. Raphael, D. (2007). Poverty and quality of life. In D. Raphael (Ed.), *Poverty and policy in Canada: Implications for health and quality of life.* Toronto: Canadian Scholars' Press Inc.

   In this chapter the author relates the quality of life implications of poverty. Drawing upon the model developed by the Centre for Health Promotion at the University of Toronto, poverty is seen as affecting all aspects of individuals' and communities' quality of life.

8. Raphael, D., Steinmetz, B., & Renwick, R. (1998). *The people, places, and priorities of Lawrence Heights/Riverdale: Findings from the community quality of life project*. Toronto: Department of Public Health Sciences. Available at www.utoronto.ca/qol/community.htm.

    These are the full reports of the community quality of life projects conducted by the Centre for Health Promotion at the University of Toronto. The themes identified by community members, service providers, and elected representatives are related to the quality of life model developed at the Centre for Health Promotion

9. Raphael, D., Steinmetz, B., & Renwick, R. (1998). *The people, places, and priorities of Lawrence Heights/Riverdale: Write-ups of the group discussions and individual interviews*. Toronto: Department of Public Health Sciences. Available at www.utoronto.ca/qol/community.htm.

    These are the detailed write-ups of the focus groups conducted as part of the community quality of life projects in Toronto. The write-ups provide the key themes identified and numerous quotations by study participants that identified these key issues.

10. Williams, A., & Kitchen, P. (2004). *Quality of life module. Quality of life in Saskatoon, SK: Achieving a healthy, sustainable community. Summary of research*. Saskatoon: University of Saskatchewan, Community-University Institute of Social Research. Available at www.usask.ca/cuisr/docs/pub_doc/quality/QoLResearchSummary2004.pdf

    The research presented in this report is part of a larger project that examines the process and results of a multi-stakeholder approach to the development and use of quality of life indicators in achieving a healthy, sustainable Saskatoon community. See also the special issue of *Social Indicators Research*, 2008, volume 85, which details this work.

RECOMMENDED WEBSITES

1. Canadian Index of Well-being (CIW)—www.atkinsonfoundation.ca/ciw

    The CIW is a partnership of national leaders, organizations, and grassroots Canadians across the country in consultation with international experts. The goal of the CIW is to provide a set of tools that will identify key indicators of health and well-being and help reshape the direction of public policy and pinpoint policy options and solutions. The result should be an improvement in the well-being of Canadians.

2. Canadian Policy Research Networks (CPRN), Quality of Life Theme—
www.cprn.com/theme.cfm?theme=15&l=en

In 1999, the CPRN began the task of creating a prototype set of national quality of life indicators to reflect a range of issues that truly matter. In 2000, 350 residents of Canada took part in 40 different dialogue groups in 21 towns and cities across Canada and discussed what mattered to them in terms of quality of life. The results of those dialogues led directly to the production of a prototype set of national quality of life indicators. The prototype consists of nine themes and 40 indicators.

3. Community Tool Kit—http://ctb.ku.edu

Located at the University of Kansas, the Community Tool Box is the world's largest resource for free information on essential skills for building healthy communities. It offers more than 7,000 pages of practical guidance on creating change and improvement, and is growing as a global resource for this work. The Community Tool Box's mission is to promote community health and development by connecting people, ideas, and resources.

4. Community Quality Improvement (CQI)—www.qualitycommunity.ca

The CQI project has taken a leading role in Sault Ste. Marie to improve community well-being. Working with community partners, CQI conducts local research in seven areas: culture/recreation, economy, education, environment, governance, health, and social well-being. Using sustainability indicators developed by the community, CQI collects quantitative and qualitative data at the local level. The community participates in discussions around the research findings to determine where they are, where they are going, and, most importantly, where they want to go.

5. Federation of Canadian Municipalities, Quality of Life Reporting System—
http://fcm.ca/english/view.asp?x=477

The Quality of Life Reporting System (QOLRS) measures, monitors, and reports on social, economic, and environmental trends in Canada's largest cities and communities. The QOLRS is a member-based initiative. Starting with 16 municipalities in 1996, the QOLRS has grown to 23 communities in seven provinces. QOLRS reports and statistics correspond to the municipal boundaries of member communities.

6. Jacksonville Community Council, Inc (JCCI)—www.jcci.org

JCCI brings people together to improve the quality of life of the community. It is world renowned for its work in developing indicators of quality of life, collecting these data, and using the findings to improve community quality of life. JCCI uses over 100 indicators in nine areas (or elements) of quality of life, including education, economy, natural environment, social environment, arts and culture, health, government, transportation, and public safety.

7. Organisation for Economic Co-operation and Development (OECD)—www. oecd.org

   The OECD is an organization of the governments of wealthy industrialized countries. It produces numerous ongoing reports, the especially important ones being *Society at a Glance*, *Health at a Glance*, and *Education at a Glance*. These reports—and others—provide up-to-date indicators of societal functioning and public policy in the service of citizens' well-being.

8. Seniors Quality of Life Project—www.utoronto.ca/seniors

   In April, 1999, the Seniors Quality of Life Project began its two-year program of research into the quality of life of seniors in seven cities across Canada. Seniors groups in Quebec City, Montreal, Ottawa, Toronto, Regina, Whitehorse, and Vancouver organized and carried out a series of public consultations on issues and factors affecting the quality of life and well-being of seniors. The goals were to: (i) collect information about the factors affecting seniors' quality of life, and (ii) develop and implement a means by which Canadian seniors in urban areas can work to influence public policies that affect their quality of life. The website contains all of the final reports and a summary report.

9. Social Planning and Research Council of BC (SPARC BC)— www.sparc.bc.ca/ resources-and-publications/category/36/community-indicators-resources

   SPARC BC is a non-partisan, charitable organization operating in BC since 1966. It focuses on social justice issues and works with communities on issues of accessibility, community development, income security, and social planning.

10. WHO—European Office: Healthy cities and urban governance—www.euro. who.int/healthy-cities

   The WHO Healthy Cities program engages local governments in health development through a process of political commitment, institutional change, capacity building, partnership-based planning, and innovative projects. It promotes comprehensive and systematic policy and planning, with a special emphasis on health inequalities and urban poverty, the needs of vulnerable groups, participatory governance, and the social, economic, and environmental determinants of health. It also strives to include health considerations in economic, regeneration, and urban development efforts.

Part III: The Role of the Social Determinants of Health

One way of considering how quality of life comes about is to examine the living circumstances to which individuals are exposed. The concept of the social determinants of health not only describes these conditions, but also suggests that attention must be paid to the public policy decisions that shape these social determinants. Nations differ profoundly in how willing the governing authorities are to support social determinants of health. Why these differences occur and their effects are the focus of this section.

Chapter 10 describes the concept of the social determinants of health and how a made-in-Canada approach to them was developed. Despite Canadian leadership in developing many related concepts, the actual implementation of these ideas in the development of public policy in Canada has fallen behind that of many other nations. Evidence concerning the importance of addressing the social determinants of health is presented, and some of the potent barriers to their being applied in the development of public policy are considered.

Chapter 11 reviews the current status of theory and research concerning the social determinants of health. It provides an overview of current conceptualizations and evidence on the impact of various social determinants of health. The contributions of different disciplines to the concept are acknowledged, but profound gaps persist in our understanding of the forces that drive the quality of various social determinants of health and why research is too infrequently translated into action. The areas of inquiry needed to help translate knowledge into action are identified.

Chapter 12 places the concept of the social determinants of health in the context of varying forms of the welfare state in modern developed nations. Canada, like the USA and the UK, is identified as a liberal welfare state in which government intervention in the workings of the marketplace is minimized. Government reluctance to offer public policies to strengthen the social determinants of health in Canada is contrasted with the situation in social democratic welfare states such as Denmark, Finland, Norway, and Sweden. Means are provided by which governmental reluctance to strengthen the social determinants of health can be countered.

Chapter 13 details how Canada, the UK, the USA, and Sweden address health promotion. The USA provides an example of little policy activity and little action in addressing the social determinants of health. Canadian authorities are more advanced in considering these issues, but there is rather little to show for it in terms of actual policy implementation. The UK is distinguished by a range of governmental activity to reduce health inequalities. Sweden, however, provides a situation where both public policy activity and actual and successful policy implementation in the service of promoting health are apparent.

CHAPTER 10

Bridging the Gap between Research Findings and Public Policy

Dennis Raphael

INTRODUCTION

In late 2002, 400 social and health policy experts, community representatives, and health researchers from Canada met at York University in Toronto at a conference entitled "Social Determinants of Health Across the Life-Span" to consider the state of ten key social determinants of health across Canada, explore the implications of these conditions for the health of Canadians, and outline policy directions to strengthen these social determinants of health. At the same time, Roy Romanow's *Building on Values: The Future of Health Care in Canada* was released. Despite submissions to the Commission that stressed the importance of the social determinants of health for the health of the population and maintaining the sustainability of the health care system, there was nary a mention of these issues in the Commission's final report, in contrast with Michael Kirby's report, *The Health of Canadians—The Federal Role*, released earlier. In this article I will outline why the social determinants of health are so important and consider reasons for the continuing gap between what is known about the social determinants of population health and governmental action on these issues. I will provide examples of nations that have incorporated thinking about social determinants of health into national policy directions.

SOCIAL DETERMINANTS OF HEALTH

While there has been profound improvement in health in industrialized nations over the past century, wide disparities in population health continue to exist between nations and among citizens within nations. Some analysts hypothesize that access to improved medical care is responsible for such differences, but best estimates are that only 10–15 percent of increased longevity since 1900 is due to improved care. More recently, differences in lifestyle behaviours such as tobacco use, diet and physical activity have been presented as the prime determinants of health. But studies conducted as early as the mid 1970s, which have been reinforced by numerous more recent studies, find these risk factors account for only a small proportion of variation in incidence among individuals in heart disease, cancers, and diabetes. There are additional factors that predict health and illness. What are these?

Nonmedical and non-lifestyle factors that affect health go by a variety of titles. The "Ottawa Charter for Health Promotion" identifies the prerequisites for health as being peace, shelter, education, food, income, a stable ecosystem, sustainable resources, social justice, and equity. Health Canada accepted direction from the Canadian Institute for Advanced Research in outlining determinants of health, many of which are societal determinants. The determinants it came up with are income and social status, social support networks, education, employment and working conditions, physical and social environments, biology and genetic endowment, personal health practices and coping skills, healthy child development, and health services.

A World Health Organization working group more recently identified ten social determinants of health: the social [class health] gradient, stress, early life, social exclusion, work, unemployment, social support, addiction, food, and transport. The organizers of the York University "Social Determinants of Health" conference synthesized these formulations to identify ten key social determinants of health that are especially relevant to Canadians: early life, education, employment and working conditions, food security, health care services, housing, income and its distribution, the social safety net, social exclusion, and unemployment and employment security.

The evidence that these social determinants of health are of more importance to the health of Canadians than biomedical and lifestyle factors is clear. As one example, adverse socio-economic circumstances during childhood are repeatedly found to be more potent predictors of the incidence of cardiovascular disease and diabetes than later life circumstances and lifestyle behaviours, facts not touched upon by the Romanow, Kirby or Manzankowski reports. The weight of the evidence indicates that social determinants of health 1) have a direct impact on health of individuals and populations, 2) are the best predictors of individual and population health, 3) structure lifestyle choices, and 4) interact with each other to produce health.

Canadian policy-makers should be aware of these findings. Canada has been a world leader in developing the implications of these findings through the health promotion and population health concepts. In 1974 the federal government's report, *A New Perspective on the Health of Canadians* (the Lalonde report), saw health and illness as being determined by human biology, environment, lifestyle, and health care organization. The document was important in that it identified determinants of health other than the health care system.

Another Canadian government document, *Achieving Health for All: A Framework for Health Promotion* (the Epp report, 1986), identified a prime goal of reducing inequities between income groups by influencing the social determinants of health when it stated that "all policies with a direct bearing on health need to be co-ordinated. The list of policy areas is long and includes, among others, income security, employment, education, housing, business, agriculture, transportation, justice, and technology." The 1999 Health Canada document, *Taking Action on Population Health: A Position Paper For Health Promotion and Programs Branch Staff*, states:

> There is strong evidence indicating that factors outside the health care system significantly affect health. These "determinants of health" include income and social status, social support networks, education, employment and working conditions, physical environments, social environments, biology and genetic endowment, personal health practices and coping skills, healthy child development, health services, gender and culture.

In spite of this accumulated knowledge, Canadians continue to be told—with some notable exceptions—by governments, health care providers, disease associations, public health units, and media that lifestyle choices are both a threat to and the salvation of their health. What is not mentioned is that the evidence for this is contested and that biomedical interventions and lifestyle choices are a small factor in whether individuals stay healthy or become ill. Not surprisingly, research indicates that the Canadian public has little awareness of the importance of the social determinants of health.

GOVERNMENT INACTION

The reasons for governmental inaction on the social determinants of health are relatively easy to ascertain but much more difficult to redress. In the context of building healthy public policy to influence the social determinants of health, the Kirby report discusses the difficulties of implementing policies requiring intersectoral action as well as longer time frames to assess effectiveness. Social determinants of health thinking require various ministries to co-ordinate policy-making and implementation.

In addition to organizational issues related to governmental functioning, policy discussions on the importance of nonmedical and non-lifestyle determinants of health are increasingly rare. Indeed, in its submission to the Romanow Commission, the Canadian Population Health Initiative (CPHI) of the Canadian Institute for Health Information commented that:

> [In] recent years, as the costs and delivery of health care have dominated the public dialogue, there has been inadequate policy development reflecting these understandings [on determinants of health]. In fact, Canada has fallen behind countries such as the United Kingdom and Sweden and even some jurisdictions in the United States in applying the population health knowledge base that has been largely developed in Canada.

The policy vacuum on social determinants of health exists within a broader context. The decline of the social welfare state in Canada and elsewhere—described by Gary Teeple in *Globalization and the Decline of Social Reform* (2000)—is driving neoliberal approaches to federal and provincial policy-making that fundamentally conflict with strengthening the social determinants of health.

Teeple argues that forces that led to the development of the welfare state at the end of World War II, and in the process strengthened the social determinants of health, were strong national identities, the need to rebuild Western economies, the strength of labour unions within national labour boundaries, the perceived threat of socialist alternatives, and a consensus for political compromise to avoid economic cycles of boom and bust. These forces led to more equitable distribution of income and wealth through social, economic, and political reforms such as progressive tax structures, social programs. and governmental structures that mitigated conflicts between business and labour, among others.

These forces are now in decline. Since the early 1970s, a fundamental change has occurred in national and global economies. The rise of transnational corporations that easily shift investments across the globe serves to pressure nations into acceding to their demands for changes that reverse reforms associated with the welfare state, thereby reducing labour costs and maximizing profits.

Indeed, government policy-making in Canada seems intent on weakening the social determinants of health. Federal program spending as a percentage of GDP is now at 1950s levels, and government policies have increased income and wealth inequalities, created crises in housing and food security, and increased the precariousness of employment.

Political pressure on federal, provincial, and local governments to conform to these shifting ideological sands blends well with the persistent bias of health workers in favour of individualistic, biomedical, and lifestyle approaches to health. The media also prefers easy-to-understand biomedical and lifestyle headlines. The social determinants of health approach is lost among such ideological imperatives.

In 1991 we, as Canadians, were profoundly healthier than were our neighbours to the south. But since then, there have been profound changes in the distribution of income and other policy domains in Canada that are directly relevant to the social determinants of health. Recent health indicators are mixed with an increase in death rates from diabetes and mental illness among Canadians, while deaths from cardiovascular disease continue to decline.

The Romanow Commission report repeats the contested notion that the lifestyle factors of tobacco use, diet, and physical inactivity—what UK sociologist Sarah Nettleton calls the "holy trinity of risk"—are the main causes of chronic disease in Canada. Only a few paragraphs are devoted to broader determinants of health. Recommendations for promoting health naively exhort governments to support Canadians in making healthy lifestyle choices.

The Romanow Commission report (unlike the Kirby report) neglects to stress the important issue of developing a strategy for developing healthy public policy to strengthen various social determinants of health. Indeed, in calling for the establishment of a Canadian Health Council, the report fails to mention any role for it in coordinating and supporting government action to address the social determinants of health.

TOWARDS THE FUTURE

The Kirby report has an excellent presentation of what is known about the importance of the social determinants of health. It recognizes that the burden of disease would be reduced by building public policy to support health determinants. While repeating the contested notion that lifestyle issues are the leading causes of chronic disease in Canada—ignoring the effects of material deprivation associated with living in absolute and relative poverty; psycho-social stress associated with income, food, and housing insecurity; and adopting unhealthy behaviours as a means of coping with such distress—the report states: "As a first step, all policies and programs established by the federal government should be assessed in terms of their impact on the health status of Canadians. A follow-up report ... will set out its findings and recommendations on the potential for, and the implications of, healthy public policy in Canada."

Participants in the "Social Determinants of Health Across the Life-Span" conference in Toronto—as part of its Toronto Charter for a Healthy Canada—stated that:

> The federal government should establish a Social Determinants of Health Task Force to consider the findings and work to implement the implications of the material presented at this Conference. The Task Force would operate to identify and advocate for policies to support population health by all levels of governmental operation.

The follow-up Kirby report on developing healthy public policy should call for such a mechanism.

But, is a healthy national public policy possible in Canada? The simple answer is yes. Nations such as Sweden and Finland are not as wealthy as Canada but have, for years, systematically incorporated thinking about the social determinants of health into their national policy agendas.

The current National Swedish Health Policy contains numerous action areas to improve population health. These activities are the responsibility of the National Institute of Public Health. The six main strategies outlined are:

- *Increase social capital in the Swedish society.* This includes efforts to decrease social inequality, counteract discrimination of minority groups, and promote local democracy.
- *Promote better working conditions.* The most important issues are to decrease long-term negative stress, promote employees' influence at work, and achieve more flexible working hours.
- *Improve conditions for children and young people.* Improve social support for families with children. Support and strengthen health-promoting schools.
- *Improve the physical environment.* Co-ordinate the work for sustainable environment with the struggle for improved health.
- *Promote healthy lifestyles.* Solidarity with those who are most vulnerable to lifestyle risks.
- *Provide good structural conditions for public health work at all societal levels.* Support to, and co-ordination of, research and education in public health science.

"In summary, the Swedish public health goals are relatively few and their structure is not very sophisticated compared with other countries. However, there are two significant qualitative aspects of the Swedish policy that may be of interest: 1) The targets are formulated in terms of the determinants of health, and 2) very thorough work has been carried out in order to achieve consensus of and raise political support for the targets. The preliminary strategies and goals are supported by five of six political parties in the Swedish parliament."

In the Swedish case study included in *Reducing Inequalities in Health: A European Perspective* (2002), Burström, Diderichsen, Östlin and Östergren point out that:

> For many years Sweden has pursued equality-oriented health and social policies, active labour market policies and family-oriented policies that have resulted in higher levels of work-place participation, less income inequality, lower poverty rates and smaller socioeconomic inequalities in the distribution of poverty than in most other countries.

The result, as expected, is that "Compared to many other countries, Sweden has low mortality rates, high life expectancy, and favourable health indicators across all socioeconomic groups."

In *Strategies for Social Protection 2010* (2001), the Finnish Ministry of Social Affairs and Health outlines preventive social policy that 1) supports growth and development of children and young people, 2) prevents exclusion, 3) supports personal initiative and involvement among the unemployed, and 4) promotes basic security in housing. Population health can be promoted and social exclusion reduced by:

- Improving efficiency and co-operation among primary, specialized and occupational health care organizations
- Providing support for the general functional capacity of people of differing ages
- Promoting lifelong learning
- Promoting well-being at work
- Increasing gender equality and social protection, which provides an incentive to work
- Giving priority to preventive policy, early intervention and actions to interrupt long-term unemployment
- Reducing regional welfare gaps
- Promoting multiculturalism
- Controlling substance abuse
- Promoting active participation in international policy-making
- Providing adequate income security as the key to building social cohesion

It should be noted that as early as 1986, four general targets were set for the population's health under the Health for All program: Adding years to life, through a decline in premature deaths; adding health to life, by showing a decline in chronic diseases, accidents, and other health problems; adding life to years, by promoting good health and functional capacity for longer in life, with welfare to match; and reducing health disparities between population groups, producing smaller health differences between genders, socio-economic categories, and people living in different regions.

The Finnish *Government Resolution on the Health 2015 Public Health Programme* (2001) concluded that progress had been made on all four goals. Life expectancy for women had risen six years since the beginning of the 1970s and that for men about seven. Infant mortality continues to be well below the EU average. Mortality rates among the over-65s have also declined considerably. Incidence of heart attacks, strokes, hypertension, rheumatoid arthritis, and many infectious diseases has fallen. Dental caries have decreased substantially, especially among young people. The percentage of under-55s on disability pension has also declined. Research shows that Finns in general, and especially middle-aged and older people, feel healthier on average than peers in the 1970s. Finally, mortality differences between the genders and different parts of the country have lessened.

CONCLUSIONS

Canadian policy-makers have repeatedly stated their commitment to maintaining and improving the health of Canadians and sustaining the health care system. Supporting the social determinants of health is an important means of doing so. Alternative approaches to promoting healthy lifestyle choices and increasing spending on medical care are unlikely to accomplish these goals in the absence of actions focused on these broader policy issues. Policy-makers should be aware of these facts. It is time for governments to act upon these social determinants of health or else to inform Canadians as to the reasons why they are unwilling to do so.

CHAPTER 11

Present Status, Unanswered Questions, and Future Directions

Dennis Raphael

INTRODUCTION

It has become commonplace among population health researchers to acknowledge that the health of individuals and populations is strongly influenced by various social determinants of health (1, 2). It is less common for health researchers to acknowledge that the quality of these social determinants of health is influenced by the organization of societies and how these societies distribute material resources among their members (3–5). And it is even less common for researchers to consider the political, economic, and social forces that shape the organizational and distributional practices of societies (6–9).

The recent publication of two texts focused on social determinants of health (1, 2) and the establishment of a World Health Organization commission on the social determinants of health (10) should not disguise the fact that the idea that societal factors are important determinants of health is not new. During the 19th century, Rudolf Virchow and Friedrich Engels outlined the political, economic, and social forces that threaten health and well-being and spawn disease and early death (11, 12).

WHAT ARE SOCIAL DETERMINANTS OF HEALTH?

The term "social determinants of health" grew out of the search by researchers to identify the specific mechanisms by which members of different socio-economic groups come to experience varying degrees of health and illness.

Another stimulus to investigating social determinants of health was the finding of national differences in population health. For example, the health status of Britons and Americans—on indicators such as life expectancy, infant mortality, and death by childhood injury rates—compares unfavorably with that of citizens in many industrialized nations (13, 14). In contrast, the health status of Scandinavians is generally superior to that seen in most nations (15, 16).

Approaches to the Social Determinants of Health

A variety of approaches to the social determinants of health exist, and all of these are concerned with the organization and distribution of economic and social resources. The 1986 *Ottawa Charter for Health Promotion* (17) identified the *prerequisites for health* as peace, shelter, education, food, income, a stable ecosystem, sustainable resources, social justice, and equity.

A British working group charged with the specific task of identifying *social determinants of health* named the social (class health) gradient, stress, early life, social exclusion, work, unemployment, social support, addiction, food, and transport (18).

A synthesis of these works identified 11 key *social determinants of health*: Aboriginal status, early life, education, employment and working conditions, food security, health care services, housing, income and its distribution, social safety net, social exclusion, and unemployment and employment security (2). This framework is important since the determinants are specifically linked to policy areas common to governmental organization of ministries and departments (19).

WHAT IS THE EVIDENCE ON THE SOCIAL DETERMINANTS OF HEALTH?

A robust body of evidence documents the importance of various social determinants of health.

Primary Determinants of Improved Health Since 1900

Profound improvements in health status have occurred in industrialized nations since 1900. Most analysts conclude that improvements in health are due to the improving material conditions of everyday life related to early childhood, education, food processing and availability, health and social services, housing, and other social determinants of health (20–23).

Primary Determinants of Health Inequalities among Citizens

Despite dramatic improvements in health in general, significant inequalities in health among citizens persist in developed nations (24, 25). These health differences result primarily from experiences of qualitatively different environments associated with the social determinants of health (26). Socio-economic position, for example, is especially important as it serves as a marker of different experiences with many social determinants of health (27).

Primary Determinants of Health Differences among Nations

Once a nation achieves a basic level of prosperity, differences in social determinants of health such as income and its distribution, quality of early childhood, and employment and working conditions explain differences in life expectancy and infant mortality rates among citizens (13).

EMERGING THEMES IN THE STUDY OF SOCIAL DETERMINANTS OF HEALTH

Three themes are emerging in social determinants of health research.

Social Determinants and Health: Dominant Frameworks

Recent theoretical thinking considers how social determinants of health "get under the skin" to influence health.

MATERIALIST APPROACH: CONDITIONS OF LIVING AS DETERMINANTS OF HEALTH

Individuals experience varying degrees of positive and negative exposures over their lives that accumulate to produce adult health outcomes (28). Material conditions—reflecting the impact of various social determinants of health—determine health by influencing the quality of individual development, family life and interaction, and community environments (29, 30).

Material conditions of life lead to differences in psychosocial stress (31, 32) that weaken the immune system and lead to increased insulin resistance, greater incidence of lipid and clotting disorders, and other biomedical insults that are precursors to adult disease (32).

Adoption of health-threatening behaviours is a response to material deprivation and stress (33). Environments determine whether individuals take up tobacco, use alcohol, have poor diets, and engage in physical activity (34).

NEOMATERIALIST APPROACH: CONDITIONS OF LIVING AND SOCIAL INFRASTRUCTURE AS DETERMINANTS OF HEALTH

Differences in health among nations, regions, and cities are related to how economic and other resources are distributed within the population (35).

Canada, for example, has a smaller proportion of lower-income people, a smaller gap between rich and poor, and spends relatively more on public infrastructure than the United States (36). Not surprisingly, Canadians enjoy better health than Americans as measured by infant mortality rates, life expectancy, and mortality from childhood injuries (37). Neither nation does as well as Sweden, where distribution of resources is much more egalitarian, low-income rates are very low, and health indicators are among the best in the world (38).

The neomaterialist view directs attention to both the effects of living conditions on individuals' health and the societal factors that determine the quality of the social determinants of health. How a society decides to distribute resources among its citizens is an especially important contributor to the quality of various social determinants of health.

PSYCHOSOCIAL COMPARISON APPROACH: HIERARCHY AND SOCIAL DISTANCE AS DETERMINANTS OF HEALTH

Health inequalities in developed nations, it is argued, are strongly influenced by citizens' interpretations of their standing in the social hierarchy (39, 40). There are two mechanisms by which this occurs.

At the individual level, the perception and experience of personal status in unequal societies lead to stress and poor health. At the communal level, widening and strengthening of hierarchy weakens social cohesion—a determinant of health.

There is an active debate concerning the relevance of each approach for understanding the health-related effects of various social determinants of health (41–43). The bulk of content of the two texts (1, 2) specifically focused on the social determinants of health takes a clear materialist position. A tremendous amount of empirical evidence has documented how social determinants of health such as income, housing, food, security, availability of health and social services, and quality of early childhood, among others, seem to act through material pathways to influence health (24, 41, 43–45). Evidence for the role of psychosocial comparison processes, however, is lacking (46). Thus the balance of evidence supports materialist and neomaterialist analyses of how social determinants influence health (41, 43).

The Importance of a Life-course Perspective

Hertzman (47) outlines three health effects relevant to a life-course perspective. *Latent effects* are biological or developmental, early life experiences that influence health later in life. Low birth weight, for instance, is a reliable predictor of incidence of adult-onset diabetes and cardiovascular disease in later life. Nutritional deprivation during childhood has lasting health effects.

Pathway effects are experiences that set individuals onto trajectories that influence health, well-being, and competence over the life course. As one example, children who enter school with delayed vocabulary are set upon a path that leads to lower educational expectations, poor employment prospects, and greater likelihood of illness and disease across the life span. Deprivation associated with poor-quality neighbourhoods, schools, and housing sets children off on paths leading to poor health status (27).

Cumulative effects represent the accumulation of advantage or disadvantage over time that manifests itself in poor health. These involve the combination of latent and pathway effects. Adopting a life-course perspective directs attention to how social determinants of health operate at every level of development—early childhood, childhood, adolescence, and adulthood—both to immediately influence health and to provide the basis for health or illness later in life.

The Importance of Policy Environments

The quality of many social determinants of health is determined by approaches to public policy. Policy issues influence the provision of adequate income, family-friendly labor policies, active employment policies involving training and support, provision of social safety nets, and the degree to which health and social services and other resources are available to citizens (48, 49–58).

Public policy decisions made by governments are driven by a variety of political, economic, and social forces (14, 59–61). Interestingly, the role of public policy in the quality of various social determinants of health is neglected by many population health researchers (62).

WHAT AREAS OF INQUIRY ARE NEEDED?

There are some key areas that could benefit from inquiry that uses a social determinants of health framework.

Recovery from illness and rehabilitation. While it is well established that social determinants of health are excellent predictors of illness and diseases, we know little about how these same health determinants lead to recovery from illness.

Concept representation and the media. There has been virtually no penetration into the media of the social determinants of health (63). What barriers prevent reporters' understanding of, and reporting on, the social determinants of health?

Public understanding and action. Given the media's coverage of health, we should not be surprised to find that the public has little understanding of the social determinants of health (64). A recent Canadian report found little public awareness of the importance of income, early childhood development, and social environments in influencing health (65). Yet, polls consistently show that many if not most citizens in Canada and the United Kingdom, for example, favor reductions in poverty and income inequality, reductions in homelessness and food bank use, and increased program spending to improve people's quality of life (28, 66). How can citizens' values be applied to influence government policy-making?

REFERENCES

1. Marmot, M., and Wilkinson, R. G. *Social Determinants of Health.* Oxford University Press, Oxford, 2000.

2. Raphael, D. (ed.). *Social Determinants of Health: Canadian Perspectives.* Canadian Scholars' Press, Toronto, 2004.

3. Esping-Andersen, G. *The Three Worlds of Welfare Capitalism.* Princeton University Press, Princeton, NJ, 1990.

4. Esping-Andersen, G. *Social Foundations of Post-Industrial Economies.* Oxford University Press, New York, 1999.

5. Esping-Andersen, G. (ed.). *Why We Need a New Welfare State.* Oxford University Press, Oxford, 2002.

6. Navarro, V. (ed.). *The Political Economy of Social Inequalities: Consequences for Health and Quality of Life.* Baywood, Amityville, NY, 2002.

7. Navarro, V. (ed.). *The Political and Social Contexts of Health.* Baywood, Amityville, NY, 2004.

8. Navarro, V., and Muntaner, C. (eds.). *Political and Economic Determinants of Population Health and Well-being: Controversies and Developments.* Baywood, Amityville, NY, 2004.

9. Bryant, T. Politics, public policy and population health. In *Staying Alive: Critical Perspectives on Health, Illness, and Health Care,* ed. D. Raphael et al. Canadian Scholars' Press, Toronto, 2006.

10. World Health Organization. *WHO to Establish Commission on Social Determinants of Health.* Geneva, 2004.

11. Virchow, R. *Collected Essays on Public Health and Epidemiology.* Science History Publications, Cambridge, UK, 1985 (1848).

12. Engels, F. *The Condition of the Working Class in England*. Penguin Classics, New York, 1987 (1845).

13. Navarro, V., et al. The importance of the political and the social in explaining mortality differentials among the countries of the OECD, 1950–1998. In *The Political and Social Contexts of Health*, ed. V. Navarro. Baywood, Arnityville, NY, 2004.

14. Raphael, D. A society in decline: The social, economic, and political determinants of health inequalities in the USA. In *Health and Social Justice: A Reader on Politics, Ideology, and Inequity in the Distribution of Disease*, ed. R. Hofrichter. Jossey Bass, San Francisco, 2003.

15. Burström, B., et al. Sweden. In *Reducing Inequalities in Health: A European Perspective*, ed. J. Mackenbach and M. Bakker. Routledge, London, 2002.

16. Vagero, D., and Lundberg, O. Health inequalities in Britain and Sweden. *Lancet* 2:35–36, 1989.

17. World Health Organization. *Ottawa Charter for Health Promotion*. World Health Organization, European Office, Geneva, 1986.

18. Wilkinson, R. G., and Marmot, M. *Social Determinants of Health: The Solid Facts*. World Health Organization, European Office, Copenhagen, 2003.

19. Raphael, D., Bryant, T., and Curry-Stevens, A. Toronto Charter outlines future health policy directions for Canada and elsewhere. *Health Promotion Int.* 19:269–273, 2004.

20. Evans, R. G., Barer, M. L., and Marmor, T. R. (eds.). *Why Are Some People Healthy and Others Not? The Determinants of Health of Populations*. Aldine DeGruyter, New York, 1994.

21. Evans, R. D. *Interpreting and Addressing Inequalities in Health: From Black to Acheson to Blair to ...* Office of Health Economics, London, 2002.

22. Davey Smith, G., Dorling, D., and Shaw, M. (eds.). *Poverty, Inequality and Health in Britain: 1800-2000: A Reader*. Policy Press, Bristol, UK, 2001.

23. Davey Smith, G., and Gordon, D. Poverty across the life-course and health. In *Tackling Inequalities: Where Are We Now and What Can Be Done?*, ed. C. Pantazis and D. Gordon. Policy Press, Bristol, UK, 2000.

24. Gordon, D., et al. *Inequalities in Health: The Evidence Presented to the Independent Inquiry into Inequalities in Health*. Policy Press, Bristol, UK, 1999.

25. Wilkins, R., Berthelot, J.-M., and Ng, E. Trends in mortality by neighbourhood income in urban Canada from 1971 to 1996. *Health Rep.* 13(suppl.):1–28, 2002.

26. Raphael, D. Introduction to the social determinants of health. In *Social Determinants of Health: Canadian Perspectives*, ed. D. Raphael. Canadian Scholars' Press, Toronto, 2004.

27. Lynch, J., and Kaplan, G. A. Socioeconomic position. In *Social Epidemiology*, ed. L. F. Berkman, and I. Kawachi. Oxford University Press, New York, 2000.

28. Shaw, M. et al. *The Widening Gap: Health Inequalities and Policy in Britain.* Policy Press, Bristol, UK, 1999.

29. Shaw, M., Dotling, D., and Mitchell, R. *Health, Place and Society.* Prentice Hall, Harlow, UK, 2002.

30. Gordon, D., and Townsend, P. (eds.). *Breadline Europe: The Measurement of Poverty.* Policy Press, Bristol, UK 2000.

31. Brunner, E., and Marmot, M. G. Social organization, stress, and health. In *Social Determinants of Health*, ed. M. G. Marmot and R. G. Wilkinson. Oxford University Press, Oxford, 1999.

32. Stansfeld, S. A., and Marmot, M. (eds.). *Stress and the Heart: Psychosocial Pathways to Coronary Heart Disease.* BMJ Books, London, 2002.

33. Jarvis, M. J. and Wardle, J. Social patterning of individual health behaviours: The ease of cigarette smoking. In *Social Determinants of Health*, ed. M. G. Marmot and R. G. Wilkinson. Oxford University Press, Oxford, 1999.

34. Raphael, D., Anstice, S., and Raine, K. The social determinants of the incidence and management of type 2 diabetes mellitus: Are we prepared to rethink our questions and redirect our research activities? *Leadership in Health Services* 16:10-20, 2003.

35. Lynch, J. W., et al. Income inequality and mortality: Importance to health of individual income, psychosocial environment, or material conditions. *BMJ* 320:1220-1224, 2000.

36. Ross, N., et al. Relation between income inequality and mortality in Canada and in the United States: Cross sectional assessment using census data and vital statistics. *BMJ* 320:898-902, 2000.

37. Sanmartin, C., and Ng, E. *Joint Canada/United States Survey of Health, 2002-03.* Statistics Canada, Ottawa, 2004.

38. Raphael, D. Addressing the social determinants of health in Canada: Bridging the gap between research findings and public policy. *Policy Options* 24(3):35-40, 2003.

39. Wilkinson, R. G. *The Impact of Inequality: How to Make Sick Societies Healthier.* New Press, New York, 2005.

40. Kawachi, I., and Kennedy, B. *The Health of Nations: Why Inequality Is Harmful to Your Health.* New Press, New York, 2002.

41. Lynch, J., et al. Is income inequality a determinant of population health? Part 1. A systematic review. *Milbank Q.* 82(1):5-99, 2004.

42. Judge, K. Income distribution and life expectancy: A critical appraisal. *BMJ* 311:1282-1285, 1995.

43. Lynch, J., et al. Is income inequality a determinant of population health? Part 2. U.S. national and regional trends in income inequality and age- and cause-specific mortality. *Milbank Q.* 82(2):355–400, 2004.

44. Acheson, D. *Independent Inquiry into Inequalities in Health.* Stationery Office, London, 1988.

45. Leon, D., and Walt, G. (eds.). *Poverty, Inequality and Health: An International Perspective.* Oxford University Press, Oxford, 2001.

46. Muntaner, C. Commentary: Social capital, social class, and the slow progress of psychosocial epidemiology. *Int. J. Epidemiol.* 33(4):1–7, 2004.

47. Hertzman, C. The case for an early childhood development strategy. *Isuma,* Autumn, 2000, pp. 11–18.

48. Auger, N., et al. Income and health in Canada. In *Social Determinants of Health: Canadian Perspectives,* ed. D. Raphael. Canadian Scholars' Press, Toronto, 2004.

49. Armstrong, P. Health, social policy, social economies, and the voluntary sector. In *Social Determinants of Health: Canadian Perspectives,* ed. D. Raphael. Canadian Scholars' Press, Toronto, 2004.

50. Browne, G. Early childhood education and health. In *Social Determinants of Health: Canadian Perspectives,* ed. D. Raphael. Canadian Scholars' Press, Toronto, 2004.

51. Bryant, T. Housing and health. In *Social Determinants of Health: Canadian Perspectives,* ed. D. Raphael. Canadian Scholars' Press, Toronto, 2004.

52. Curry-Stevens, A. Income and income distribution. In *Social Determinants of Health: Canadian Perspectives,* ed. D. Raphael. Canadian Scholars' Press, Toronto, 2004.

53. Friendly, M. Early childhood education and care. In *Social Determinants of Health: Canadian Perspectives.* ed. D. Raphael. Canadian Scholars' Press, Toronto, 2004.

54. Galabuzi, G. F. Social exclusion. In *Social Determinants of Health: Canadian Perspectives,* ed. D. Raphael. Canadian Scholars' Press, Toronto, 2004.

55. Jackson, A. The unhealthy Canadian workplace. In *Social Determinants of Health: Canadian Perspectives,* ed. D. Raphael. Canadian Scholars' Press, Toronto, 2004.

56. Shah, C. Aboriginal health. In *Social Determinants of Health: Canadian Perspectives,* ed. D. Raphael. Canadian Scholars' Press, Toronto, 2004.

57. Shapcott, M. Housing. In *Social Determinants of Health: Canadian Perspectives,* ed. D. Raphael. Canadian Scholars' Press, Toronto, 2004.

58. Tremblay, D. G. Unemployment and the labour market. In *Social Determinants of Health: Canadian Perspectives,* ed. D. Raphael. Canadian Scholars' Press, Toronto, 2004.

59. Hofrichter, R. The politics of health inequities: Contested terrain. In *Health and Social Justice: A Reader on Politics, Ideology, and Inequity in the Distribution of Disease.* Jossey Bass, San Francisco, 2003.

60. Raphael, D, and Bryant, T. Maintaining population health in a period of welfare state decline: Political economy as the missing dimension in health promotion theory and practice. *Promot Educ.* 13(4):236–242, 2006.

61. Raphael, D. Towards the future: Policy and community actions to promote population health. In *Health and Social Justice: A Reader on Politics, Ideology, and Inequity in the Distribution Of Disease*, ed. R. Hofrichter. Jossey Bass, San Francisco, 2003.

62. Bambra, C., Fox, D., and Scott-Samuel, A. Towards a politics of health. *Health Promotion Int.* 20(2):187–193, 2005.

63. Hayes, M. Media Suffering from "Tunnel Vision," Says Health Researcher. Simon Fraser University, Burnaby, B.C., 2002.

64. Eyles, J., et al. What determines health? To where should we shift resources? Attitudes towards the determinants of health among multiple stakeholder groups in Prince Edward Island, Canada. *Soc. Sci. Med.* 53(12):1611–1619, 2001.

65. Canadian Population Health Initiative. *Select Highlights on Public Views of the Determinants of Health.* Ottawa, 2005.

66. Adams, M. *Fire and Ice: The United States, Canada and the Myth of Converging Values.* Penguin Books Canada, Toronto, 2003.

CHAPTER 12
Maintaining Population Health in a Period of Welfare State Decline

Dennis Raphael and Toba Bryant

INTRODUCTION

There is increasing recognition in the health promotion and population health fields that the primary determinants of health lie outside the health care and behavioural risk arenas. Decisions made by governments in sectors such as income distribution, social security, education, and housing—summed up in the phrase social determinants of health—are prime contributors to the realization of health. These decisions—which in their entirety may be considered as reflecting commitments to the welfare state—are heavily influenced by politics. Yet, there has been a neglect of the politics of health.

In Canada, there is little explicit acknowledgment by health promoters and population health researchers of the importance of the politics of health. We analyze the role played by politics in determining health by considering the forces behind recent public policy decisions that impact upon the social determinants of health.

REVIEWING HEALTH PROMOTION AND POPULATION HEALTH

Health promotion as outlined by the World Health Organization represents a commitment to improve health and well-being through societal change (MacDonald & Davies, 1998).

In line with its predominantly structural approach to promoting health, the Ottawa Charter for Health Promotion outlined the basic prerequisites for health—or social determinants of health in modern usage—of peace, shelter, education, food, income, a stable ecosystem, sustainable resources, social justice, and equity (World Health Organization, 1986). One of the five pillars of health promotion action is building healthy public policy.

Population health concepts focus upon the role societal factors play in determining the health of populations (Evans, Barer, & Marmor, 1994). We would expect it to include analyses of how political, economic, and social forces shape the availability and distribution of a range of health-supporting resources—income, housing, social and health services, etc.—among societal members. Such analyses would provide a context for understanding the quality of various social determinants of health. In reality, most population health approaches place little emphasis upon political and economic forces in favour of more immediate situational issues such as social and physical environments (Raphael, 2004a).

THE SOCIAL DETERMINANTS OF HEALTH AND PUBLIC POLICY

The term *social determinants of health* grew out of the search by researchers to identify the specific exposures by which members of different socio-economic groups come to experience varying degrees of health and illness. Table 12.1 provides recent formulations of the social determinants of health. The *SDOH National Conference* list is unique in that it specifically focuses on the public policy environment (e.g., income and its distribution) rather than characteristics associated with individuals (e.g. income and social status) (Raphael, 2004a).

Public policy is important for health promotion and population health because it determines the quality of the social determinants of health. The establishment of the World Health Organization's Commission on the Social Determinants of Health underscores this emerging recognition (World Health Organization, 2004).

Table 12.1: Various Conceptualizations of the Social Determinants Of Health

Ottawa Charter[1]	Health Canada[2]	World Health Organization[3]	SDOH National Conference[4]
Peace	Income and	Social gradient	Aboriginal status
Shelter	social status	Stress	Early life
Education	Social support	Early life	Education
Food	networks	Social exclusion	Employment
Income	Education	Work	and working
Stable ecosystem	Employment	Unemployment	conditions
Sustainable	and working	Social support	Food security
resources	conditions	Addictions	Health care
Social justice	Physical	Food	services
Equity	environments	Transport	Housing
	Social		Income and its
	environments		distribution
	Healthy child		Social safety net
	development		Social exclusion
	Health services		Unemployment
	Culture		and employment
	Gender		security

1. World Health Organization, 1986; 2. Health Canada, 1998; 3. Wilkinson & Marmot, 2003; 4. Raphael et al., 2004

CANADIAN PUBLIC POLICY AND THE SOCIAL DETERMINANTS OF HEALTH

What is the nature of policy change in Canada that threatens the quality of numerous social determinants of health? The most obvious manifestation of the public policy environment is government program spending as a percentage of Gross Domestic Product (GDP). In 1992 the proportion of Canadian GDP allocated to program spending began to decline such that spending levels are now at late 1940s' levels (Hulchanski, 2002). Canadian governmental program spending as a proportion of GDP is now among the lowest of developed nations (Bryant, 2006).

Government spending is a key aspect of how societies differ in their commitment to social infrastructure and support for citizens across the life-span (Shaw, Dorling, Gordon, & Davey Smith, 1999). Such differences in spending—correlated strongly with a range of other ideological commitments—provide a context for understanding the environments in which health promotion and population health activities are situated (Navarro & Shi, 2001). The states of two key social determinants of health illustrate current policy environments in Canada: income and its distribution, and housing.

INCOME AND INCOME DISTRIBUTION

2001 Canadian census data show a disturbing picture of incidence of low income (similar to what is internationally termed the poverty rate) among Canadians (16.2% of individuals and 12.6% of families) (Statistics Canada, 2004b). The low income rate for female-led single families is 56%. The incidence of low income is especially high among residents of major Canadian urban areas, where over 20% of Vancouver families are so identified, 19% of Toronto families, and 23% of Montreal families. Two volumes provide recent analyses of where Canada stands in relation to other industrialized nations (Innocenti Research Centre, 2005; Rainwater & Smeeding, 2003).

HOUSING

Housing is an important social determinant of health. Spending excessive amounts of income on housing reduces resources available for other social determinants of health such as food and recreation (Bryant, 2004). The proportion of tenants spending >30% of total income on rent is very high in Canadian cities (43% in Vancouver, 42% in Toronto, and 36% in Montreal) (Statistics Canada, 2004a). The proportion spending >50%—putting them at risk of imminent homelessness—is also strikingly high (22% in Vancouver, 20% in Toronto, and 18% in Montreal). A significant proportion of urban dwellers (>8%) live in substandard housing.

THE POLITICS OF PUBLIC POLICY: INSIGHTS FROM POLITICAL ECONOMY

Political economy is about the relationships among the state, the economy, and civil society (Hofrichter, 2003). As an area of inquiry, it provides insights that link specific disciplines such as political science, economics, and sociology (Armstrong, Armstrong, & Coburn, 2001). The issues considered within such a perspective are the production and distribution of wealth, the relative political power of social classes that is related to issues of capital accumulation and the organization of labour, and the extent to which society relies extensively on state control of the distribution of resources versus market control of such activities (Esping-Andersen, 1985, 1990, 1999, 2002).

Critical health researchers use these concepts to argue that how a society produces and distributes societal resources among its population—that is, its political economy—are important determinants of population health (Coburn, 2000, 2004, 2006; Navarro, 2002; Navarro & Muntaner, 2004). These links become clearer as evidence accumulates of how income distribution, employment conditions, and availability of social and health services are important determinants of population health (Marmot & Wilkinson, 2006; Raphael, 2004b).

Esping-Andersen Typology of Modern Capitalist Welfare States

In spite of increasing economic globalization, nations systematically differ in their commitments to policy environments that can strengthen the social determinants of health. Esping-Andersen identified three worlds of welfare capitalism: social democratic, conservative, and liberal (Esping-Andersen, 1990, 1999). There are many differences in public policy among these types. The social democratic welfare states (Finland, Sweden, Denmark, and Norway) emphasize universal welfare rights and provide generous benefits and entitlements. The conservative welfare states (France, Germany, Spain, and Italy) also offer generous benefits, but provide these based on employment status with emphasis on male primary breadwinners. The liberal Anglo-Saxon economies (UK, USA, Canada, and Ireland) provide only modest benefits and step in only when the market fails to provide adequate supports. These liberal states depend on means-tested benefits targeted to only the least well-off.

These concepts are very useful for understanding why nations differ systematically in their commitment to strengthening the social determinants of health. Tremblay applies the typology to understand current employment policy in Canada (Tremblay, 2004), while Friendly does so in relation to Canadian approaches to early childhood education care (Friendly, 2004). Jackson considers how the typology helps explain the state of employment and working conditions in Canada (Jackson, 2004).

Findings suggest that health promoters concerned with the social determinants of health and public policies that strengthen them need to look to the nations ruled by social democratic parties for insights and ideas for promoting health. What are the political and economic forces that lead to such approaches to health and well-being?

THE BUILDING BLOCKS OF HEALTH PUBLIC POLICY AND POPULATION HEALTH

Bryant identifies the following political and economic forces that support health-enhancing public policies (Bryant, 2006):

- The ability of "left" parties to influence government decision-making. This ability is strengthened by adoption of proportional representation in the electoral process.
- High union density and the ability of unions to provide a united front in negotiating wages and employment conditions.
- Proactive governmental action in developing a range of public policies. This involves commitment to active labour policy (training, supports, and unemployment benefits), support for women's employment, adequate spending to support families, providing assistance to the unemployed and those with disabilities, and providing educational and recreational opportunities.
- Commitment to policies that reduce social exclusion and promote democratic participation.

CONCLUSION: IMPLICATIONS FOR HEALTH PROMOTION AND POPULATION HEALTH

While Canada is a liberal welfare state, members of the liberal welfare state club are not monolithic in policy approaches. Canada developed a universal health care system while the USA did not.

The UK has embarked upon a systematic policy initiative to reduce child poverty while Canada has not. Nations systematically shift their basket of public policies to become outliers within their welfare state group. This suggests room for policy action in support of health.

Advocacy is about influencing governments to enact policies in support of health. This requires that health promoters and population health researchers be more explicit concerning their analysis of the role governments play in influencing the social determinants of health. It also requires explicit recognition of the role political and economic forces play in shaping these policies and the need to confront these sources of power and influence when they threaten health and well-being. Once these forces are acknowledged, health promoters and population health researchers must go public with these conclusions to influence public policy (Raphael & Bryant, 2006).

Community-based Education and Research

At the community level citizens can be involved in these activities through a process of participatory policy research. In this approach citizens are asked to consider decisions that governments and agencies make that are influencing their health and well-being. It is similar to conventional participatory research, with the exception that the focus of community members is clearly directed towards public policy rather than local community issues.

The best means of promoting health and improving population health involves Canadians—and others—being informed about the political and economic forces that shape the health of a society. Once so empowered, they can consider political and other means of influencing these forces. Health promoters and population health researchers need to "get political" and recognize the importance of political and social action in support of health. This seems a rather daunting task, but one that holds the best hope of promoting the health of citizens in Canada and elsewhere (Bryant, Raphael & Rioux, 2006).

REFERENCES

Armstrong, P., Armstrong, H. & Coburn, D. (Eds.). (2001) *Unhealthy times: The political economy of health and care in Canada*. Oxford University Press, Toronto.

Bryant, T. (2004) "Housing and health." In Raphael, D. (Ed.) *Social determinants of health: Canadian perspectives*. Canadian Scholars Press, Toronto.

Bryant, T. (2006) "Politics, public policy and population health". In Raphael, D. Bryant, T. & Rioux, M. (Eds.) *Staying alive: Critical perspectives on health, illness, and health care*. Canadian Scholars' Press, Toronto.

Bryant, T., Raphael, D., & Rioux, M. (2006) "Towards the future—Current themes in health research and practice in Canada." In Raphael, D. Bryant, T. & Rioux, M. (Eds.), *Staying alive: Critical perspectives on health, illness, and health care*. Canadian Scholars' Press, Toronto.

Coburn, D. (2000) "Income inequality, social cohesion and the health status of populations: The role of neo-liberalism." *Social Science & Medicine* vol. 51, pp. 135–146.

Coburn, D. (2004). "Beyond the income inequality hypothesis: Globalization, neo-liberalism, and health inequalities." *Social Science & Medicine*, vol. 58, pp. 41–56.

Coburn, D. (2006) "Health and health care: A political economy perspective." In Raphael, D., Bryant, T., & Rioux, M. (Eds.) *Staying alive: Critical perspectives on health, illness, and health care*. Canadian Scholars' Press, Toronto.

Esping-Andersen, G. (1985) *Politics against markets: The social democratic road to power*. Princeton University Press, Princeton.

Esping-Andersen, G. (1990) *The three worlds of welfare capitalism*. Princeton University Press, Princeton.

Esping-Andersen, G. (1999) *Social foundations of post-industrial economies*. Oxford University Press, New York.

Esping-Andersen, G. (Ed.) (2002) *Why we need a new welfare state*. Oxford University Press, Oxford, UK.

Evans, R. G., Barer, M. L. & Marmor, T. R. (1994) *Why are some people healthy and others not?: The determinants of health of populations*. Aldine de Gruyter, New York.

Friendly, M. (2004) "Early childhood education and care." In Raphael, D. (Ed.) *Social determinants of health: Canadian perspectives*. Canadian Scholars' Press, Toronto.

Health Canada. (1998). *Taking action on population health: A position paper for health promotion and programs branch staff*. Ottawa: Heath Canada.

Hofrichter, R. (2003) "The politics of health inequities: Contested terrain." In *Health and social justice: a reader on ideology, and inequity in the distribution of disease*. Jossey Bass, San Francisco.

Hulchanski, D. J. (2002) *Can Canada afford to help cities, provide social housing, and end homelessness? Why are provincial governments doing so little?* Centre for Urban and Community Studies, University of Toronto. Viewed n.d. <http://www.tdrc.net/Report-02-07-DH.htm>

Innocenti Research Centre (2005) Child poverty in rich nations, 2005. Report card No. 6. Innocenti Research Centre, Florence. Viewed n.d. <http://www.unicef.ca/press/childpoverty/>

Jackson, A. (2004) "The unhealthy Canadian workplace." In Raphael, D. (Ed.) *Social determinants of health: Canadian perspectives.* Canadian Scholars' Press, Toronto.

MacDonald, G. & Davies, J. (1998) "Reflection and vision: Proving and improving the promotion of health." In Davies, J. & MacDonald, G. (Eds.) *Quality, evidence, and effectiveness in health promotion: Striving for certainties.* Routledge, London UK.

Marmot, M. & Wilkinson, R. (2006) *Social determinants of health* (2nd ed.) Oxford University Press, Oxford, UK.

Navarro, V. (Ed.) (2002) *The political economy of social inequalities: Consequences for health and quality of life.* Baywood Press, Amityville, NY.

Navarro, V. & Muntaner, C. (Eds.) (2004) *Political and economic determinants of population health and well-being: Controversies and developments.* Baywood Press, Amityville, NY.

Navarro, V. & Shi, L. (2001) "The political context of social inequalities and health." *Social Science & Medicine* vol. 52, pp. 481–491.

Rainwater, L. & Smeeding, T. M. (2003) *Poor kids in a rich country: America's children in comparative perspective.* Russell Sage Foundation, New York.

Raphael, D. (2004a) "Introduction to the social determinants of health." In Raphael, D. (Ed.) *Social determinants of health: Canadian perspectives.* Canadian Scholars' Press, Toronto.

Raphael, D. (Ed.) (2004b) *Social determinants of health: Canadian perspectives.* Canadian Scholars' Press, Toronto.

Raphael, D., & Bryant, T. (2006) "Public health concerns in Canada, USA, UK, and Sweden: Exploring the gaps between knowledge and action in promoting population health." In Raphael, D. Bryant, T. & Rioux, M. (Eds.) *Staying alive: critical perspectives on health, illness, and health care.* Canadian Scholars' Press, Toronto.

Shaw, M., Dorling, D., Gordon, D., & Davey Smith, G. D. (1999) The widening gap: Health inequalities and policy in Britain. The Policy Press, Bristol, UK.

Statistics Canada (2004a) *2001 community profiles for Canadian cities.* Statistics Canada, Ottawa.

Statistics Canada (2004b) *Income of Canadian families: 2000 census.* Statistics Canada, Ottawa.

Tremblay, D. G. (2004) "Unemployment and the labour market." In Raphael, D. (Ed.) *Social determinants of health: Canadian perspectives.* Canadian Scholars Press, Toronto.

Wilkinson, R., Marmot, M. (2003). *Social determinants of health: The solid facts.* Copenhagen: World Health.

World Health Organization (1986) *Ottawa charter for health promotion.* World Health Organization, European Office. Viewed n.d. <http://www.who.int/hpr/NPH/docs/ottawa_charter_hp.pdf>

World Health Organization (2004) *WHO to establish commission on social determinants of health.* World Health Organization, Geneva. Viewed n.d. <http://www.who.int/social_determinants/en/>

CHAPTER 13

The State's Role in Promoting Population Health

Dennis Raphael and Toba Bryant

INTRODUCTION

> *Public health is ultimately a question of what kind of society we wish to live in. There is a close connection between democracy participation, equality and social security on the one hand and good public health on the other* [1, p. 24].

Promoting and maintaining the public's health is an ongoing preoccupation of national, regional, and municipal governments around the globe. Promoting health comprises three distinct, though potentially related, sets of activities: (a) traditional public health activities of environmental protection, infection control, and modifying risk behaviours; (b) advocating for and contributing to developing health supporting public policy; and (c) delivering health care services [2]. The first two sets of activities—our concern in this article—are primarily concerned with promoting the health of the population, while health care services focus on treating individuals who are ill.

In Canada, these components for the most part operate independently of each other. With few exceptions, public health agencies and units carry out traditional public health activities, policy-makers design public policy in their spheres of influence, and health care professionals deliver health services through the universally accessible health care system. In the UK and Sweden, however, efforts have been made to integrate traditional public health activities with the development of health-supporting public policy. In the USA, public health authorities are frequently involved in delivering health care services to indigent populations.

In this paper we are concerned with answering these questions:

- What principles and concepts direct public health activities in each nation?
- What do local public health units do to promote health?
- To what extent are these activities integrated with the development of health-related public policy?
- What are the ideological components and antecedents of public health approaches?

CANADA

> Canada has led the world in understanding health promotion and population health ... However in recent years, as the costs and delivery of health care has dominated the public dialogue, there has been inadequate policy development reflecting these understandings. In fact, Canada has fallen behind countries such as the United Kingdom and Sweden and even some jurisdictions in the United States in applying the population health knowledge base that has been largely developed in Canada [3, p. 1].

This statement from the authoritative *Canadian Population Health Initiative* presents the contrast between Canadian public health rhetoric and action. Canada has been seen as a leader in innovative approaches to public health [4]. Canadians developed health promotion principles of equity and participation and the population health focus on determinants of health.

The 1990s saw the rhetorical emphasis upon health promotion—with its explicit concern with community engagement—eclipsed by the field of population health that focused on researching how social, economic, and physical environments influenced health [5]. Health Canada has taken the best concepts of health promotion and population health to argue for an integrated approach, the *Population Health Template*, shown as Fig. 13.1.

Public policy approaches to influence the determinants of health continue to be stressed—and generally ignored—in federal, provincial, and local public health documents, disease-oriented association mission statements, and Royal Commission and Senate Committee health reports in Canada [6,7]. As noted, however, a major Canadian health research institute sees little evidence that Canada applies its own concepts

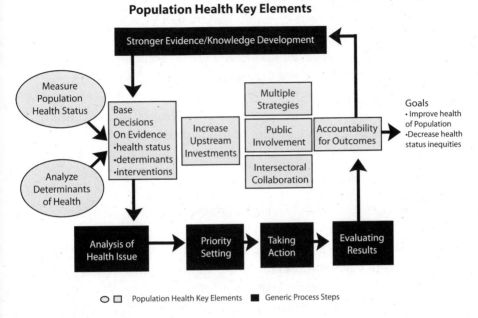

Population Health Key Elements

Fig. 13.1: Health Canada's Population Health Template

to promoting Canadians' health [3]. This conclusion has been verified by numerous analyses of the Canadian public health scene that indicate that policy approaches to addressing broader determinants of health are few and far between [8–10]. Why might this be so?

The SARS crisis of 2003—backed up by public health lobbying—increased interest in public health mandates. In response, the federal government established a National Public Health Agency that is led by a minister of state and a national health officer and staffed by former employees of Health Canada's Population and Public Health Branch. The agency consists of National Collaborating Centres for: Public Policy and Risk Assessment, Public Health Methodologies and Tools Development, Infectious Disease, Environmental Health, Aboriginal Health, and, of some note, Determinants of Health [11].

The mandate of the National Collaborating Centre for Determinants of Health is described as:

> *Working in close collaboration with researchers, the public health community, and government and non-governmental organizations in Atlantic Canada to study the role of the*

"social determinants of health"—factors such as physical and cultural isolation, income/socio-economic status, employment, immigration status, mental illness, and risk behaviours such as smoking and lack of physical activity [11].

It is too early to determine whether the extent of Agency concern will be with broader policy issues related to determinants of health or be diverted to issues of risk behaviours.

Provincial and Local Public Health Activities

Canadian public health practice is for the most part divorced from concern with modifying the broader determinants of health. Provincial health authorities direct the activities of local health unit activities and, with few exceptions (see Quebec and British Columbia's health objectives) [12,13], focus is on behavioural approaches to health promotion and population health. This is true even when provincial documents detail the importance of broader determinants of health.

An extensive survey of how local public health units across Canada addressed the issue of poverty—representing the effect of numerous broader determinants of health—found that half of 98 responding health regions did not have any initiatives addressing poverty issues. Among those that did, virtually all were dealing with the consequences of poverty rather than addressing its causes [9]. Similar findings are reported in regard to implementing broad health goals related to social issues [10].

Against the Grain: Taking Healthy Public Policy Seriously

In summary, Canadian public health activity emphasizes the traditional roles of health protection and behavioural approaches to health promotion. Health Canada, the Canadian Public Health Association, and various social welfare and social policy organizations raise issues of healthy public policy and the broader determinants of health, but there is little penetration of these concepts into public awareness or public health action. There are only isolated instances of public health action to influence healthy public policy.

UNITED STATES OF AMERICA

The current infant mortality rate of seven infant deaths per 1000 live births is moving in the wrong direction ... This ranks the United States 28th internationally. Clearly, we still have more work to do for our communities, our families, and our children [14, p. 4].

The USA has one of the worst health profiles of modern industrialized nations. It is one of the least developed welfare states, spending less than most industrialized nations on public infrastructure to support citizens. It is the only modern industrialized nation to not provide health care to citizens as a matter of course. Public health concern with broader determinants of health and developing healthy public policy to influence health is very poorly developed.

National Policy Documents and Reports

Healthy People 2010 is the USA's national public health plan and contains a large number of health objectives and enabling activities to achieve these [15]. Like other US documents it contains a chapter on the broader determinants of health and its health model is consistent with a broader health perspective (Fig. 13.2). It has a prominent emphasis on issues of access to health care, which is not surprising given that 17% or 45 million Americans are without health insurance coverage.

However, closer inspection of the document reveals the role played by broader determinants of health is undeveloped. The *Leading Health Indicators* "[R]eflect the major health concerns in the United States at the beginning of the 21st century." These objectives—physical activity, overweight and obesity, tobacco use, substance abuse, responsible sexual behavior, mental health, injury and violence, environmental quality, immunization, and access to health care—are firmly planted in the biomedical and behavioural public health model.

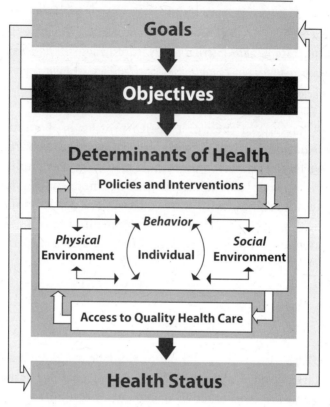

Fig. 13.2: Healthy People 2010 Model of Health Determinants.

The Institute of Medicine's *The Future of the Public's Health* has similar shortcomings [16]. It has a chapter on developments in population health, yet these concepts do not diffuse to the rest of the volume. Virtually all issues to be addressed are health-care-related or behaviourally focused around diet, tobacco use, or physical activity. Policy is conceived narrowly as legislation related to risk behaviours and health protection.

In summary, public health activity in the USA is characterized by (a) a focus on providing access to health care to its citizens; (b) a focus on ethnic and racial disparities in health rather than a range of health determinants; (c) a reluctance to consider the roles structural aspects of society, such as the distribution of economic and social resources, play in influencing health; and (d) a reluctance to identify influencing broad public policy as an appropriate focus of public health action.

UNITED KINGDOM

> A new minister for public health will attack the root causes of ill health, and so improve lives and save the [National Health Service] money. Labour will set new goals for improving the overall health of the nation, which recognise the impact that poverty, poor housing, unemployment and a polluted environment have on health [17].

The UK has a longstanding intellectual and academic concern with inequalities in health. In 1980 the *Black Report* revealed that despite a generation of accessible health care, class-related health inequalities had not only been maintained but in many instances had widened [18]. The report appeared at the onset of the conservative Thatcher era and its recommendations for promoting health were ignored for two decades. Instead, during this period, numerous policies served to widen income and health inequalities. The election of the New Labour government in 1997 saw the ongoing academic and policy concern with health inequalities translated into a government-wide effort to address health inequalities through the implementation of public policy initiatives.

In 1997, the New Labour government commissioned the *Acheson Commission into Inequalities in Health*. The commission considered a wide range of evidence and in its synopsis concluded:

> The weight of scientific evidence supports a socioeconomic explanation of health inequalities. This traces the roots of ill health to such determinants as income, education and employment as well as to the material environment and lifestyle [19].

It offered 13 sets of recommendations that spanned a range of determinants of health that include poverty, income, tax, and benefits; education; employment; housing and environment; mobility, transport, and pollution, among others. It emphasized that (a) all policies likely to have an impact on health should be evaluated in terms of their impact on health inequalities; (b) high priority should be given to the health of families with children; and (c) further steps should be taken to reduce income inequalities and improve the living standards of poor households.

Government Action Plans

Among the major policy initiatives in response to the Inquiry's findings was *Reducing Health Inequalities: An Action Report* that focused on the areas in Table 13.1 [20].

Table 13.1: Reducing Health Inequalities: The UK Agenda for Action

Upon election in 1997, the UK Labour Government organized a strategy based on nine themes. Specific policies are listed to illustrate its action approach
Raising living standards and tackling low income by introducing a minimum wage and a range of tax credits and increasing benefit levels
Education and early years by introducing policies to improve educational standards, creating 'Sure Start'—preschool services in disadvantaged areas, free to those on low incomes
Employment by creating a range of welfare-to-work schemes for different priority groups
Transport and mobility by setting targets to reduce road traffic accidents, develop safe walking and cycling routes, and standardize concessionary fares for older people
Issues for the National Health Service (NHS) include working in partnership with local authorities to tackle the wider determinants of health, reviewing the resource allocation formula to local health care agencies, developing frameworks to standardize care across the country for particular conditions, and broadening the NHS's performance framework to include fair access and improving health
Building healthy communities by investing in a range of regeneration initiatives in disadvantaged areas, including Health Action Zones
Housing by changing capital financial rules to promote investment in social housing and introducing special initiatives to tackle homelessness
Reducing crime by investing in range of community-led crime prevention schemes and tackling drug misuse
Public health issues—the first-ever Minister for Public Health oversaw a range of initiatives to encourage healthy lifestyles, strengthen the public health workforce, and tackle specific problems such as fluoridation of water supplies

Source: Adapted from Benzeval [21] England, Box 12.3. In: Mackenbach J., Bakker M. (editors), *Reducing Inequalities in Health: European Perspectives*. London UK: Routledge, p. 207.

There are some key aspects of the Agenda for Action and related documents such as *Opportunity for All Tackling Poverty and Social Exclusion* (1999), *A New Commitment to Neighbourhood Renewal: National Strategy Action Plan* (2001) and *From Vision to Reality* (2001) that contrast with the public health situation in Canada and the USA [22]. The first is the recognition that health inequalities are a cause for serious concern. The second is the serious use of available research evidence by government authorities. The third is the recognition that these areas are cause for concern not only by health ministries and departments but also the entire government. Fourth, there is a commitment to action through the development and implementation of public policy. And fifth, there is a goal for the National Health Service to promote equitable access to services in relation to need and their taking the lead in working with other agencies to tackle the broader determinants of health.

Reviews of these Initiatives

In 2003, an extensive evaluation of these initiatives concluded significant progress had been made in tackling health inequalities [23]. Evidence concerning health inequalities had been gathered, health inequalities had been placed on the policy agenda to a significant extent, and a diverse range of activities with increasing integration and coherence had been developed. Indicators of outcomes and policy implementation were beginning to emerge though impacts upon health status were not yet apparent. The authors concluded: *"Many challenges remain but the prospects for tackling inequalities are good"* (p. 52).

In summary, public health and health policy attention in the UK is directed to addressing inequalities in health. It is difficult to avoid the conclusion that "Debate on policy to inform health inequalities is alive and well in the United Kingdom" [24, p. 286].

SWEDEN

> *"Sweden and Finland are world leaders in public health. As Canada works to develop a pan-Canadian public health strategy, I look forward to learning more about public health systems around the world."* Canadian Minister of State for Public Health, Carolyn Bennett [25].

The 2001 Swedish Ministry of Health and Social Affairs document *Towards Public Health on Equal Terms* illustrates government understandings of the nature of health:

> The health of the population is affected by a range of what are known as determinants. These are factors that in part relate to the structure of society and in part to people's lifestyles and habits. The Government's work in the public health field extends to both these types of factors [26, p. 1].

The 2001 document proposes an explicit role for public health policy in reducing health inequalities between various groups in society. Policy areas identified include employment, education, agriculture, culture, transport, and housing. The January 2003 statement emphasizes promoting health and closing the major health gaps in society [27].

The 2002/2003 *Public Health Bill* outlines plans for promoting these objectives. Municipalities and county councils are to draw up and evaluate targets, and then report on these activities. National coordination of these activities is led by the Minister for Public Health and Social Services and carried out by the National Institute of Public Health. The Institute has drawn up a plan for skills development in public health work for those already working in relevant professions.

The Swedish National Institute of Public Health objectives that direct these activities focus on the "factors in society or in our living conditions that influence health" (Table 13.2). The first six objectives: "[R]elate to what are normally considered to be structural factors, i.e. conditions in society and our surroundings that can be influenced primarily by moulding public opinion and by taking political decisions on different levels." The last five "concern lifestyles which an individual can influence him/herself, but where the social environment normally plays a very important part."

Table 13.2: The 11 Target Areas of the New Swedish Public Health Policy

The Swedish Government has defined 11 target areas for all work in the field of public health
Participation and influence in society
Economic and social prerequisites
Conditions during childhood and adolescence
Health in working life
Environments and products
Health-promoting health services
Protection against communicable diseases
Sexuality and reproductive health
Physical activity
Eating habits and food
Tobacco, alcohol, illicit drugs, doping and gambling

Source: Swedish National Institute for Public Health. *Sweden's New Public Health Policy*. Stockholm: Swedish National Institute for Public Health. 2003. Online at *http://www.fhi.se/en/About-FHI/Public-health-policy/*

The Swedish health initiative is accompanied by a very detailed action agenda that mandates municipal and local involvement in identifying public health objectives consistent with the national vision of public health. It specifies steps to be taken to identify goals, provide actions to implement these, and then carry out evaluation activities to assure implementation. Such development of an elaborative infrastructure together with the commitment of virtually all political parties would seem to assure implementation of this ambitious agenda.

In summary, it is apparent that a public health approach based on the broader determinants of health is consistent with long-standing Swedish approaches to public policy [28]. Sweden implemented social welfare policies during the 1920s and the long tradition of establishing and maintaining a strong welfare state makes Swedish public health officials receptive to new developments in health promotion, population health, and the broader determinants of health.

UNDERSTANDING VARIATIONS IN PUBLIC HEALTH APPROACHES

It is difficult to avoid the conclusion that approaches to public health are driven by dominant political ideologies and long-standing approaches to public policy within jurisdictions. The accumulating evidence concerning the impact upon health and well-being of broader determinants of health is available to policy-makers in Canada, the USA, the UK, and Sweden. What is striking is the degree of variation in commitment to applying these findings across these nations.

In Canada and the USA, progressive concepts associated with health promotion and population health are inconsistent with nascent neoliberal approaches to governance that emphasize individualism rather than communal approaches to resource allocation.

In the UK, a new government came to power with an explicit commitment to deal with health inequalities through action on public policy. They established a commission whose members were oriented towards a materialist approach to promoting the public's health. Once the inquiry reported, they chose to act upon the recommendations. In Sweden, there are long-standing ideological commitments to addressing social inequalities that blends well with a broader approach to health policy. In both these cases, the presence of research evidence in support of public policy approaches to reducing health inequalities supports these policy initiatives, but are not the essential stimulus for such actions.

The ideological underpinnings of various health models and how they influence policy development have been extensively discussed [5,29–32]. Each rise of a particular government ideology—be it neo-liberal or social democratic—causes us to reflect upon these issues anew. Public health approaches are clearly related to dominant public policy approaches [28].

REFERENCES

1. Agren, G. Sweden's new public health policy: National Public Health Objectives for Sweden. Stockholm: Swedish National Institute of Public Health; 2003.

2. Turnock, B.J. Public Health: What it is and how it works. Mississauga, Canada: Jones and Bartlett Publishers; 2004.

3. Canadian Population Health Initiative. Canadian Population Health Initiative Brief to the Commission on the Future of Health Care in Canada. CPHI. Retrieved 20 February 2004, from the World Wide Web: http://secure.cihi.ca/cihiweb/en/downloads/cphi_policy_romanowbrief_e.pdf, 2002.

4. Restrepo, H.E. Introduction. In: PAH Organization (editor), Health promotion: An anthology. Washington DC: Pan American Health Organization, 1996, p. ix–xi.

5. Robertson, A. Shifting discourses on health in Canada: From health promotion to population health. Health Promotion International 1998;13:155–66.

6. Kirby, M.J. The health of Canadians: The federal role. Ottawa: Standing Senate Committee on Social Affairs, Science and Technology; 2002.

7. Romanow, R.J. Building on values: The future of health care in Canada. Saskatoon: Commission on the Future of Health Care in Canada; 2002.

8. Sutcliffe, P., Deber, R., Pasut, G. Public health in Canada: A comparative study. Canadian Journal of Public Health 1997;88:246–9.

9. Williamson, D. The role of the health sector in addressing poverty. Canadian Journal of Public Health 2001;92:178–82.

10. Williamson, D., Milligan, C.D., Kwan, B., Frankish, C.J., Ratner, P.A. Implementation of provincial/territorial health goals in Canada. Health Policy 2003;64:173–91.

11. Government of Canada. Government of Canada announces National Collaborating Centre for Determinants of Health. Public Health Agency. Retrieved 14 September 2005, from the World Wide Web, 2004.

12. Government of British Columbia. A report on the health of British Columbians. Victoria, Canada: Government of British Columbia, 2000.

13. Government of Quebec. Goals of the Ministry of Health and Social Services. Ministry of Health and Social services. Retrieved 12 September 2005, from the World Wide Web.

14. Howse, J., Caldwell, M.C. The state of infant health: Is there trouble ahead? In: United Health Foundation (editor), America's health: state health rankings. Seattle WA: United Health Foundation, 2004.

15. U.S. Department of Health and Human Services. Healthy people 2010: Understanding and improving health. Washington DC: U.S. Department of Health and Human Services, 2000.

16. Institute of Medicine. The future of the public's health in the 21st century. Washington DC: National Academies Press, 2002.

17. UK Labour Party. New Labour because Britain deserves better. UK Labour Party. Retrieved from the World Wide Web: http://www.psr.keele.ac.uk/area/uk/man/lab97.htm, 1997.

18. Black, D., Smith, C. The Black report. In: Townsend, P. Davidson, N. Whitehead, M. editors. Inequalities in health: The Black report and the health divide. New York: Penguin; 1992.

19. Acheson, D. Independent inquiry into inequalities in health. Stationary Office. Retrieved from the World Wide Web: http://www.official-documents.co.uk/document/doh/ih/contents.htm, 1998.

20. Department of Health. Reducing health inequalities: An action report. London UK: Department of Health, 1999.

21. Benzeval, M. England. In: Mackenbach, J., Bakker, M., editors. Reducing inequalities in health: A European perspectives. London UK: Routledge; 2002.

22. Department of Health. Publications from the Department of Health. Department of Health. Retrieved 30 January 2005, from the World Wide Web: http://www.dh.gov.uk/Home/fs/en., 2004.

23. Exworthy, M., Stuart, M., Blane, D., Marmot, M. Tackling health inequalities since the Acheson inquiry. Bristol, UK: Policy Press; 2003.

24. Oliver, A. Nutbeam, D. Addressing health inequalities in the United Kingdom: A case study. Journal of Public Health Medicine 2003;25:281–7.

25. Health Canada. Minister Carolyn Bennett and Chief Public Health Officer of Canada participate in launch of European Public Health Agency. Health Canada. Retrieved from the World Wide Web, 2004.

26. Swedish Ministry of Health and Social Affairs. Towards public health on equal terms. Stockholm, Sweden: Swedish Ministry of Health and Social Affairs, 2001.

27. Swedish Ministry of Health and Social Affairs. Public health objectives. Stockholm, Sweden: Swedish Ministry of Health and Social Affairs, 2003.

28. Bryant, T. Politics, public policy and population health. In: Raphael, D. Bryant, T. Rioux, M. editors. Staying alive: Critical perspectives on health, illness, and health care. Toronto: Canadian Scholars Press; 2006.

29. Labonte, R. Health promotion and empowerment: Practice frameworks. Toronto: Centre for Health Promotion and ParticipACTION; 1993.

30. Seedhouse, D. Health: The foundations of achievement. New York: John Wiley and Sons; 2003.

31. Tesh, S. Hidden arguments: Political ideology and disease prevention policy. New Brunswick, NJ: Rutgers University Press; 1990.

32. Williams, G., Popay, J. Social science and the future of population health. In: Jones, L., Sidell, M. editors. The challenge of promoting health. London UK: The Open University; 1997, p. 260-73.

RECOMMENDED READINGS

1. Gasher, M., Hayes, M., Ross, I., Hackett, R., Gutstein, D., & Dunn, J. (2007). Spreading the news: Social determinants of health reportage in Canadian daily newspapers. *Canadian Journal of Communication, 32*(3), 557–574.
This article reports on a series of formal interviews with English-language and French-language health reporters. The study found that Canadian health reporters overemphasize health care issues and personal health habits as the expense of the role of social determinants. The comments of reporters are quite telling.

2. Graham, H. (2004). Social determinants and their unequal distribution: Clarifying policy understandings. *Milbank Quarterly, 82*(1), 101–124.
The author makes the distinction between social determinants of health and the distribution of the social determinants of health. Graham argues that the social factors promoting and undermining the health of individuals and populations—the social determinants of health—should not be confused with the social processes—social inequalities that create their unequal distribution. More emphasis needs to be placed on social inequalities for a determinants-oriented approach to be effective.

3. Irwin, A. & Scali, E. (2007) Action on the social determinants of health: An historical perspective. *Global Public Health, 2*(3), 235–256.
This article reviews public health action on social determinants over the past five decades. The historical record highlights the problems health

policy approaches incorporating social determinants face from entrenched interests. The authors argue that advocates need to build political support for action by developing collaborative relationships with policymakers.

4. Labonte, R., & Schrecker, T. (2007). Globalization and social determinants of health: Introduction and methodological background. Part 1 of 3. *Globalization and Health, 3*(5).

 Labonte, R., & Schrecker, T. (2007). Globalization and social determinants of health: The role of the global marketplace. Part 2 of 3. *Globalization and Health, 3*(6).

 Labonte, R., & Schrecker, T. (2007). Globalization and social determinants of health: Promoting health equity in global governance. Part 3 of 3. *Globalization and Health, 3*(7).

 These three articles provide groundbreaking analyses of how economic globalization is affecting the quality of the social determinants of health and what can be done about it.

5. Marmot, M., & Wilkinson, R. (2006). *Social determinants of health*, 2nd ed. Oxford, UK: Oxford University Press.

 This UK book is an important contribution to the debate about the determinants of health. It clearly lays out the importance of non-medical and non-behavioural factors upon health. While it has a broad focus, it is primarily concerned with UK and European developments. Like many health sciences books it tends to de-politicize health issues and downplay public policy issues.

6. Raphael, D. (ed.). (2008). *Social determinants of health: Canadian perspectives*, 2nd ed. Toronto, ON: Canadian Scholars' Press Inc.

 This volume updates and extends the analysis of the state of various social determinants of health in Canada contained in the first edition. This work represents a unique undertaking in the social determinants of health area in that it brings together those working in early childhood education and care, education and literacy, employment and working conditions, food security, gender, health services, housing, income and its distribution, social exclusion, the social safety net, and unemployment and job insecurity with those specifically focused on the health effects of these issues.

7. Raphael, D., Anstice, S., & Raine, K. (2003). The social determinants of the incidence and management of type 2 diabetes mellitus: Are we prepared to rethink our questions and redirect our research activities? *Leadership in Health Services, 16*, 10–20.

 This article applies the social determinants of health concept to understand the role of social determinants in type II (adult-onset) diabetes. These kinds of analyses are rarely done and the paper suggests the value of such an approach for promoting health.

8. Raphael, D., & Farrell, E.S. (2002). Beyond medicine and lifestyle: Addressing the societal determinants of cardiovascular disease in North America. *Leadership in Health Services, 15*, 1–5.

This article brings together a range of research that indicates how important the social determinants of health concept is for understanding cardiovascular disease.

9. Starfield, B. (2007). Pathways of influence on equity in health. *Social Science and Medicine 64*, 1355–1362.

This article reviews some of the different pathways by which social determinants of health influence health. The author focuses on explicating the societal factors—particularly social inequalities and societal institutions—that lead to health inequalities.

10. Commission on the Social Determinants of Health (2008). *Closing the gap in a generation: Health equity through action on the social determinants of health.* Geneva: World Health Organization.

The Final Report of the Commission sets out key areas of daily living conditions and of the underlying structural drivers that influence them in which action is needed. It provides analysis of social determinants of health and concrete examples of types of action that have proven effective in improving health and health equity in countries at all levels of socioeconomic development.

RECOMMENDED WEBSITES

1. Baywood Publishing Company—www.baywood.com

Baywood publishes important books on the determinants of health. It also publishes the *International Journal of Health Services*, which contains cutting-edge articles on the social determinants of health and the political determinants of health, as well as analysis of health care issues from a critical perspective.

2. Canadian Senate Sub-Committee on Population Health—http://tinyurl.com/ypwhhq

The mandate of this sub-committee is to examine and report on the impact of the multiple factors and conditions that contribute to the health of Canada's population—known collectively as the social determinants of health. The sub-committee website provides transcripts of expert testimony and a number of reports on the quality of the social determinants of health and what needs to be done in Canada to improve their quality.

3. International Commission on the Social Determinants of Health—www.who.int/social_determinants

The International Commission on Social Determinants of Health supports countries and global health partners to address the social factors leading to ill health and inequities. It draws the attention of society to the social determinants of health that are known to be among the primary causes of poor health and inequalities between and within countries. The determinants include unemployment, unsafe workplaces, urban slums, globalization, and lack of access to health systems.

4. International Society for Equity in Health—www.iseqh.org

The purpose of this society is to promote equity in health and health services internationally through education, research, publication, communication, and charitable support.

5. Luxembourg Income Study (LIS)—www.lisproject.org

The LIS is a cross-national data archive located in Luxembourg. It produces numerous working papers that document how public policies shape income distribution among citizens. Many of the papers are comparative analyses of how nations differ in distributing income and wealth and creating or reducing poverty.

6. National Coordinating Centre for the Determinants of Health (NCCDH)—www.nccdh.ca

NCCDH focuses on the social and economic factors that influence the health of Canadians. Its role is to engage researchers, policy-makers, health practitioners, and the public so as to better include knowledge about the broad determinants of health in policy and practice decisions that will achieve social justice and health for all.

7. Organisation for Economic Co-operation and Development (OECD)—www.oecd.org

OECD is an organization of governments of the wealthy industrialized countries. It produces numerous ongoing reports, the especially important ones being *Society at a Glance*, *Health at a Glance*, and *Education at a Glance*. These reports—and others—provide up-to-date indicators of societal functioning and public policy in the service of citizens' well-being.

8. Policy Press—www.policypress.org.uk

The Policy Press is a leading social science publisher of books, reports, and journals. Based at the University of Bristol, it publishes on a wide range of subjects including social policy and social welfare, family policy, social work, public policy, criminal justice, and housing and urban policy. Many of its titles are multi- and cross-disciplinary.

9. Politics of Health Group (PoHG)—www.pohg.org.uk

PoHG consists of people who believe that power exercised through politics and its impact on public policy is of fundamental importance for health. PoHG believes that: (i) the opportunity for good health is the fundamental human right; and (ii) it is the responsibility of governments to strive for equitable social, economic, and environmental conditions in which the health of all can thrive.

10. The Townsend Centre for International Poverty Research—www.bris.ac.uk/poverty.

The Townsend Centre was established in response to the United Nations First International Decade for the Eradication of Poverty (1997–2006) and in recognition of the work of Professor Peter Townsend. The governments of the world have committed themselves, through the United Nations and the OECD, to the goal of eradicating poverty by the end of the 21st century. The university sector can support this goal by providing high-quality interdisciplinary research into effective anti-poverty policies

Part IV: Vulnerable Populations

Particular groups in Canada are more vulnerable to experiencing poorer quality of life. Part IV provides information about the quality of life of different racial groups, Aboriginal Canadians, persons with disabilities, and women. Why these groups appear to be more vulnerable is described and policy options to remedy these situations are presented.

Chapter 14 examines the situation of Indigenous populations in Canada, the USA, Australia, and New Zealand. It adapts the Human Development Index (HDI) to examine how the broad social, economic, and health statuses of Indigenous populations in these countries have changed since 1990. Between 1990 and 2000, the HDI scores of Indigenous peoples in North America and New Zealand improved at a faster rate than those of the general population, closing the gap somewhat in human development.

Chapter 15 considers the employment opportunities and outcomes of different racial groups in Canada. Its review of employment income data and labour market shows that as compared to Canadians of European descent, during the last census period racialized groups and recent immigrants both showed a double-digit income gap, higher unemployment, lower participation rates, and concentrations in low-income occupations.

Chapter 16 is a summary of some of the findings of a report entitled *Supports and Services for Adults and Children Aged 5–14 with Disabilities in Canada*. It examines the requirements and unmet needs for employment supports and services. The longer report from which this is taken was commissioned by the Federal-Provincial-Territorial Ministers Responsible for Social Services and released on December 3, 2004.

Chapter 17 is a call by the Council of Canadians with Disabilities and the Canadian Association for Community Living for the federal government to take leadership in combatting the poverty and exclusion of Canadians with disabilities. The document provides data on the situations of persons with disabilities in Canada and detailed descriptions for policy action.

Chapter 18 provides gender-equality indicators that were developed in conjunction with Status of Women Canada to measure the balance of the experiences of Canadian women and men in three domains: income, work, and learning. As has been the case in the past, significant issues remain in achieving gender equity in a number of domains in Canada.

CHAPTER 14

Indigenous Well-being in Four Countries

Martin Cooke, Francis Mitrou, David Lawrence, Eric Guimond, and Dan Beavon

BACKGROUND

As of January, 2007, we were two years into the second United Nations International Decade of the World's Indigenous Peoples. This may be a surprise, as this type of pronouncement of the importance of the rights and equality of the world's Indigenous peoples tends to capture media attention for only a short time before fading from the headlines. The average conditions of Indigenous peoples are generally well below national levels and disparities between Indigenous and non-Indigenous populations in health, social, and economic outcomes exist worldwide, in rich and poor countries alike, despite widely differing geographic, historical, and cultural contexts [1,2]. Among highly developed countries, Canada, the United States, Australia, and New Zealand are often seen as natural comparators in terms of Indigenous well-being. These countries consistently place near the top of the United Nations Development Programme's *Human Development Index (HDI)* rankings, yet all have minority Indigenous populations with much poorer health and social conditions than their non-Indigenous compatriots [3]. First Nations (Registered non-status Indians), Métis, and Inuit in Canada, Australian Aboriginal and Torres Strait Islander peoples, New Zealand Māori, and American Indians and Alaska Natives in the United States have each been subjected to the loss of culture, paternal protectionism, and occasional violence that have characterized Indigenous-settler state relations in these former British colonies [4,5].

In this paper we examine how the broad social, economic, and health statuses of Indigenous populations in these countries have changed since the 1990s, using an adaptation of the United Nations Human Development Index (HDI).

METHODS

The Human Development Index

The United Nations Development Program (UNDP)'s HDI has been used since 1990 to compare countries in terms of "human development," defined as the enlargement of choices made possible by education and literacy, a decent material standard of living, and a long and healthy life. Health is measured using life expectancy, knowledge is measured via educational participation and adult literacy rates, and the material standard of living is captured by GDP per capita, reported in Purchasing Power Parity (PPP) dollars. These three indicators are combined, with equal weighting, to give an overall HDI score.

RESULTS AND DISCUSSION

Population Size

The United States has the largest Indigenous population, estimated at 4,119,300 in the 2000 Census. However, American Indians and Alaska Natives comprise only 1.5 percent of the total American population. In relative terms, the Māori population is the largest, accounting for 14 percent of the total New Zealand population (at 526,200 people in the 2001 Census). Just over 2 percent of Australians (or 410,000 people) identified as being Aboriginal or Torres Strait Islander people in the 2001 Census. In Canada, 976,301 people or 3.3 percent of residents self-identified as Aboriginal in the 2001 Census.

Life Expectancy

Improvements in Indigenous life expectancy and in closing the gap between Indigenous and non-Indigenous peoples have varied among these four countries. The national life expectancy estimates for the total population of each of the four countries in question was over 75 years throughout the 1990/1–2000/1 decade. Figure 14.1

shows life expectancy at birth, from official estimates, for the four Indigenous populations of these countries over the same 10-year period. Canadian Registered Indians had the highest life expectancy of all of these populations, rising from 70.6 years to 72.9 years. Māori life expectancy also improved, from 69.4 years in 1996 to 71.1 years in 2001.

In Canada, the life expectancy gap reduced from 7.3 to 5.8 years over the decade. At the end of the period, the gap in life expectancy between Māori and non-Māori New Zealanders had declined only slightly, if at all, to 8.5 years in 2001. Australian Aboriginal people and Torres Strait Islanders stand out for having the lowest life expectancy, at 59.6 years in both 1991 and 2001. As life expectancy for non-Aboriginal Australians rose, the gap to Aboriginal people increased from 20.6 years to 23.2 years. American Indians and Alaska Natives began the period with a life expectancy of 70.2 years. This rose to 71.1 years in 1995/6, but fell again to 70.6 years in 2001, increasing the gap between Indigenous and non-Indigenous Americans from 5.2 years to 6.0 years (Table 14.1).

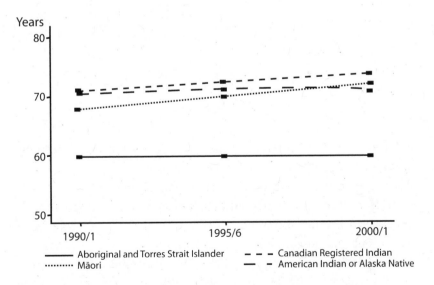

Fig. 14.1: Life Expectancy at Birth, 1990/1–2000/1.

Table 14.1: Life Expectancy at Birth, Years (Life Expectancy Index Score)

	Australia Non-Aboriginal	Aboriginal and Torres Strait Islander	Gap
1990/1	80.2 (.920)	59.6 (.577)	20.6 (.343)
1995/6	81.4 (.939)	59.4 (.573)	22.0 (.366)
2000/1	82.8 (.964)	59.6 (.576)	23.2 (.388)
	Canada Non-Aboriginal	Canadian Aboriginal (Registered Indian)	Gap
1990/1	77.9 (.882)	70.6 (.760)	7.3 (.122)
1995/6	78.5 (.892)	72.2 (.787)	6.3 (.105)
2000/1	78.7 (.895)	72.9 (.798)	5.8 (.097)
	New Zealand Non-Aboriginal	Māori	Gap
1990/1	76.4 (.856)	67.7 (.712)	8.7 (.144)
1995/6	78.0 (.883)	69.4 (.741)	8.6 (.142)
2000/1	79.6 (.910)	71.1 (.769)	8.5 (.141)
	United States Non-Aboriginal	American Indian and Alaska Native	Gap
1990/1	75.4 (.841)	70.2 (.753)	5.2 (0.88)
1995/6	76.2 (.854)	71.1 (.768)	5.1 (.086)
2000/1	76.6 (.859)	70.6 (.760)	6.0 (.099)

Educational Attainment

Progress in educational attainment was slightly more evident. Figure 14.2 presents the Educational Attainment Index for the Indigenous and non-Indigenous populations in these countries. In the first panel, the consistent improvement in educational attainment for Māori is most striking, narrowing the gap with non-Māori. Although there was a smaller difference in educational attainment between Indigenous and non-Indigenous Australians, there is no evidence of this gap closing. Although the educational attainment of Aboriginal and Torres Strait Islanders increased, it did not keep pace with the improvements in the non-Indigenous population. The result was a slight widening of the gap in educational attainment.

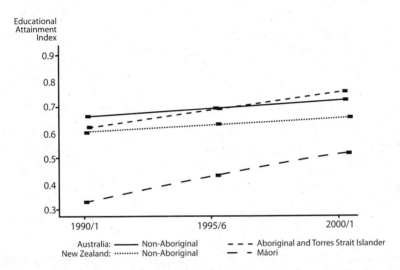

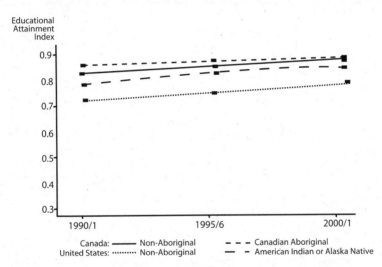

Figure 14.2: Education Attainment Index Scores, 1990/1–2000/1.

Education attainment index scores, 1990/1–2000/1.

Educational attainment scores were generally higher among North American populations. In the United States, the gap in the Educational Attainment Index was the smallest, and fell from 1990 to 2000. In Canada, the gap also narrowed between 1991 and 2001.

Table 14.2 shows how the educational attainment index is derived from the two component measures. In general, all four countries had high values on the adult literacy proxy measures, and the gaps between

Indigenous and non-Indigenous populations improved between 1991 and 2001. The Māori population had the lowest proportion aged 15 and over with some basic school qualification, at about 57 percent in 2001, and the largest gaps between Indigenous and non-Indigenous people. However, these gaps declined considerably between 1991 and 2001, from 29 to 20 percentage points. In 2001, 83% of the Australian Aboriginal population 15 and older had attained primary school or higher. The Canadian Indigenous population scored somewhat higher, and the American Indian and Alaska Native population had the highest adult literacy proxy scores, at 0.91 in 2001.

Table 14.2: Educational Attainment Proxy Measures

Country	Adult Literacy Proxy	Gross Enrolment Proxy
Australia	1991, 1996: Proportion 15 and older that left school aged 15 years or older. 2001: Proportion 15 or older with highest educational qualification year 9 or higher.	1991, 1996: Proportion of those 18–24 still in school or left school aged 18 or older. 2001: Proportion of those 18–24 still in school, or with highest educational qualification year 12 or equivalent.
Canada	Proportion 15 and older with grade nine or higher educational attainment.	Proportion of those 18–24 with secondary school certificate, some college, trades, or technical, or university.
New Zealand	Proportion aged 15 and older with no school qualification.	Proportion aged 18–24 with sixth form or higher qualification.
United States	Proportion aged 15 and older with grade nine or higher educational attainment.	Proportion aged 18–24 with high-school graduation, GED, or higher educational attainment.

Table 14.3 presents the proportion of the population aged 18–24 with high-school or higher education, our measure of educational participation. The attainment of all of the Indigenous populations improved considerably over the decade. However, in Australia and New Zealand this improvement did not keep pace with the increasing educational attainment among the non-Indigenous populations, and these countries saw the gaps widen between Indigenous and non-Indigenous populations.

Table 14.3: Educational Attainment Measures, 1990/1–2000/1

	Adult Literacy Proxy (2/3 weight)			Gross Enrolment Proxy (1/3 weight)			Educational Attainment Index		
	Non-Aboriginal	Aboriginal	Gap	Non-Aboriginal	Aboriginal	Gap	Non-Aboriginal	Aboriginal	Gap
Australia Aboriginal and Torres Strait Islander									
1991	0.85	0.84	0.02	0.28	0.13	0.15	.659	.598	.061
1996	0.86	0.84	0.02	0.33	0.17	0.16	.686	.618	.068
2001	0.88	0.86	0.02	0.38	0.22	0.16	.713	.644	.069
2001 *	0.91	0.83	0.07	0.69	0.31	0.38	.832	.659	.176
Canada Aboriginal									
1991	0.86	0.82	0.05	0.76	0.51	0.25	.826	.713	.113
1996	0.88	0.85	0.03	0.77	0.53	0.24	.843	.738	.105
2001	0.90	0.88	0.02	0.79	0.56	0.23	.866	.773	.093
New Zealand Māori									
1991	0.65	0.35	0.29	0.54	0.27	0.28	.611	.325	.286
1996	0.70	0.45	0.25	0.63	0.37	0.27	.674	.421	.253
2001	0.78	0.57	0.20	0.67	0.38	0.29	.741	.508	.233
American Indian and Alaska Native									
1990	0.90	0.88	0.03	0.77	0.63	0.13	.857	.795	.062
2000	0.92	0.91	0.02	0.75	0.67	0.08	.863	.827	.036

Note: Australian 1991–2001 figures are calculated using age at school-leaving.

* 2001 figures are calculated using educational attainment.

Median Income

Although the educational attainment of Indigenous people increased over the decade, real incomes tended to fall over the 1990–2000 period. Median annual incomes from all sources for those aged 15 and over with income are presented in year 2000 Purchasing Power Parity dollars in Table 14.4. In Australia, Canada, and New Zealand, real median incomes fell for the Indigenous and non-Indigenous populations between 1990 and 2000. In Canada and New Zealand, incomes fell between 1990 and 1995, rising somewhat thereafter, whereas Australian median incomes declined even more steeply between 1995 and 2001.

Figure 14.3 presents the income index, calculated using median individual income. In all of these countries, the gap in income index scores between Indigenous and non-Indigenous citizens fell. In Canada, the effect of an economic recession in the early 1990s seems to have been greater for non-Indigenous than Indigenous Canadians, probably because of greater attachment to the labour force. The gap in income fell from PPP$11,114 to PPP$8,904 between 1990 and 2000, and the gap in income index scores fell from 0.074 to 0.065. In the United States the gap also fell, from PPP$6,724 to PPP$5,050 in median income, and from 0.071 to 0.046 in terms of the income index.

Table 14.4: Median Annual Income, 2000 PPP$ (Income Index Score)

	Australia Non-Aboriginal	Aboriginal and Torres Strait Islander	Gap
1990/1	25,795 (.927)	16,283 (.850)	9,512 (.077)
1995/6	25,579 (.925)	15,337 (.840)	10,242 (.085)
2000/1	21,767 (.898)	12,268 (.803)	9,499 (.095)
	Canada Non-Aboriginal	Canadian Total Aboriginal	Gap
1990/1	31,084 (.958)	19,970 (.884)	11,114 (.074)
1995/6	26,441 (.931)	16,931 (.857)	9,410 (.074)
2000/1	27,617 (.938)	18,713 (.873)	8,904 (.065)
	New Zealand Non-Aboriginal	Māori	Gap
1990/1	30,973 (.957)	23,936 (.914)	7,037 (.043)
1995/6	29,020 (.946)	22,838 (.906)	6,182 (.040)
2000/1	29,756 (.951)	23,024 (.908)	6,732 (.043)
	United States Non-Aboriginal	American Indian and Alaska Native	Gap
1990/1	19,372 (.879)	12,648 (.808)	6,724 (.071)
2000/1	21,050 (.893)	16,000 (.847)	5,050 (.046)

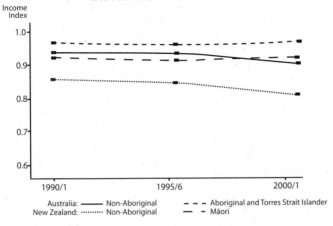

Australia: —— Non-Aboriginal   — — — Aboriginal and Torres Strait Islander
New Zealand: ·········· Non-Aboriginal   — — Māori

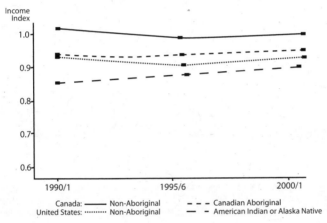

Canada: —— Non-Aboriginal   — — — Canadian Aboriginal
United States: ·········· Non-Aboriginal   — — American Indian or Alaska Native

Figure 14.3: Income Index Scores, 1990/1–2000/1.

Progress was again uneven in Australia. Over the 1990 to 2000 period, median incomes for both Indigenous and non-Indigenous Australians and New Zealanders declined. The difference between non-Aboriginal Australians and Aboriginal and Torres Strait Islanders was PPP$9,512 in 1990, rising to PPP$10,242 in 1995 and decreasing again to PPP$9,499 by 2000. Despite the fact that the gap in median income was the same at the beginning and end of the decade, the lower median income for both populations resulted in an increasing gap when calculated according to the discounted income index formula. In New Zealand, where the gap between Māori and non-Māori incomes is smaller, the income index gap was the same at the beginning and end of the period.

Indigenous Human Development Index Scores

Following the methodology described earlier, these three indices—life expectancy, educational attainment, and income—are combined into a single HDI measure. Examining the trends in HDI scores, we see that the trends are somewhat different in these countries (Table 14.5). The HDI scores of American and Canadian Indigenous populations increased over the 1990 to 2000 decade at a faster rate than the non-Indigenous populations, closing the gap in human development. The difference between non-Indigenous and Indigenous Canadians fell from 0.103 in 1991 to 0.085 in 2001. In the United States, the gap decline was sharper, from 0.074 to 0.061 by 2000.

Māori HDI scores also improved at a faster rate than non-Māori New Zealanders'. The improvement in Māori HDI scores from 0.650 in 1991 to 0.728 in 2001 means a decrease in the HDI gap.

Table 14.5: Aboriginal Human Development Index Scores 1991–2001

	Australia Non-Aboriginal	Aboriginal and Torres Strait Islander	Gap
1990/1	.835	.675	.160
1995/6	.850	.677	.173
2000/1	.858	.674	.184
	Canada Non-Aboriginal	**Canadian Aboriginal**	**Gap**
1990/1	.889	.786	.103
1995/6	.889	.794	.095
2000/1	.900	.815	.085
	New Zealand Non-Aboriginal	**Māori**	**Gap**
1990/1	.808	.650	.158
1995/6	.835	.689	.146
2000/1	.867	.728	.139
	United States Non-Aboriginal	**American Indian and Alaska Native**	**Gap**
1990/1	.859	.785	.074
2000/1	.872	.811	.061

Note: Australian 2001 figures calculated using extrapolated educational attainment (see text).

While the gaps between Indigenous and non-Indigenous populations in these three countries closed over the decade, Australia stands out for a relative lack of progress on these indicators (Figure 14.4). The HDI score for Aboriginal and Torres Strait Islanders decreased slightly over the period, while the scores for non-Aboriginal Australians improved. The result is a widening gap in HDI scores, from 0.160 in 1990 to 0.184 by 2001.

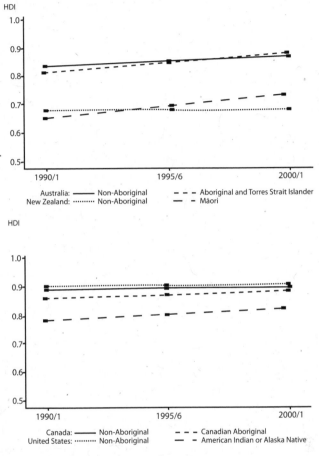

Figure 14.4:Human Development Index Scores, 1990/1–2000/1.

Indigenous Populations—An International Perspective

These Indigenous HDI scores can be used to calculate positions for the four Indigenous populations in question among the countries ranked in the UNDP's 2003 *Human Development Report* (which also uses 2001 data) [3]. As described above, the measures used by the UNDP are not available for these populations. In order to make our figures closely comparable to the UNDP's measure, we adjusted each of our measures by the ratio of the UNDP's measure for the national population to our measure for the national population. Under the assumption that the ratio between, for example, the UNDP's adult literacy rate and our own census measure holds for both the Indigenous and non-Indigenous populations, we can use that ratio to estimate an HDI score for these Indigenous populations that is comparable to the countries in the *Human Development Index*.

As Table 14.6 shows, each of these four countries was well within the group of nations that the UNDP identifies as having "high human development." By 2001, the American Indian and Alaska Native population and the Canadian Indigenous population had joined these countries, with HDI scores comparable to South Korea or the Czech Republic and Belarus or Trinidad and Tobago, respectively. By 2001, Māori would rank around 73rd among nations in the HDI league tables, among those countries with "medium" levels of human development. Australian Aboriginal and Torres Strait Islander peoples would rank approximately 104th, comparable to China and Cape Verde in terms of HDI score. This would also be classified among countries having "medium" levels of human development.

CONCLUSION

It is acknowledged that these measures give only a very rough assessment of the degree to which the well-being of Indigenous peoples in these countries has improved. They necessarily hide a great deal of heterogeneity among these populations, and omit many other aspects of well-being or "human development." However, these simple indicators of life expectancy, educational attainment, and median income do give us a picture of the overall health and socioeconomic status of these populations, and how they have changed over the 1990s.

The resulting picture is best described as one of inconsistent progress. The improvement in overall HDI scores for Indigenous peoples in Canada, New Zealand, and the United States is good news, but the lack of progress in Australia is worrying. Furthermore, even in those countries in which the relative well-being of Indigenous populations did improve, as judged by their HDI scores, the gaps on some indicators widened in some years. This suggests that further improvements in the social, economic, and physical health of Indigenous peoples cannot be taken for granted, and that further efforts must be made if we are to see these gaps close further by the end of this decade.

Table 14.6: Selected International and Aboriginal HDI Scores, 2001

HDI Rank	Country	HDI Score
	Selected Countries with High Human Development (0.800–1)	
1	Norway	.944
2	Iceland	.942
3	Sweden	.941
4	*Australia*	.939
5	Netherlands	.938
6	Belgium	.937
7	*United States*	.937
8	*Canada*	.937
9	Japan	.932
13	United Kingdom	.930
16	Austria	.929
17	France	.925
19	Spain	.925
20	*New Zealand*	.917
23	Portugal	.896
30	Republic of Korea	.879
	U.S. American Indian and Alaska Native	.877
32	Czech Republic	.861
	Canadian Aboriginal Population	.851
34	Argentina	.849
42	Costa Rica	.831
43	Chile	.831
52	Cuba	.806
53	Belarus	.804
54	Trinidad and Tobago	.802
55	Mexico	.800
Selected Countries with Medium Human Development (0.500–0.799)		
73	Saudi Arabia	.769
	New Zealand Māori	.767
75	Ukraine	.766
85	Philippines	.751
94	Dominican Republic	.737
103	Cape Verde	.727
	Australian Aboriginal and Torres Strait Islanders	.724
104	China	.721
105	El Salvador	.719
120	Egypt	.648
Selected Countries with Low Human Development (0.–0.499)		
142	Cameroon	0.499
150	Haiti	0.467
161	Côte d'Ivoire	0.396

Source: UNDP (2003); authors' calculations.

REFERENCES

1. Eversole, R.: Overview: Patterns of Indigenous disadvantage worldwide. In *Indigenous peoples and poverty: An international perspective*. Edited by: Eversole, R., McNeish JA, Cimadamore AD. London: Zed Books; 2005:29–37.

2. Stephens, C., Porter, J., Nettleton, C., Willis, R.: Disappearing, displaced, and undervalued: A call to action for Indigenous health worldwide. *Lancet* 2006, 367:2019–28.

3. United Nations Development Program: *Human development report 2003*. New York: Oxford University Press; 2003.

4. Armitage, A.: *Comparing the policy of Aboriginal assimilation: Australia, Canada, and New Zealand*. Vancouver: UBC Press; 1995.

5. Cornell, S.: Indigenous jurisdiction and daily life: Evidence from North America. *Paper presented at the national forum on Indigenous health and the treaty debate 2004* [http://www.gtcentre.unsw.edu.au/publications/papers/docs/2005/6 StephenCornell.pdf]. University of New South Wales, Sydney.

FURTHER READING

Ajwani, S., Blakely, T., Robson, B., Bonne, M., Tobias, M.: Decades of Disparity: Ethnic mortality trends in New Zealand 1980–1999. Wellington: New Zealand Ministry of Health; 2003.

Alwaji, S., Blakely, T., Robson, B., Atkinson, J., Kiro, C.: Unlocking the numerator-denominator bias III: adjustment ratios by ethnicity for 1981–1999 mortality data. The New Zealand Census-Mortality Study. *N Z Med J* 2003, 116(1175):U456.

Australian Bureau of Statistics: 1996 census of population and housing: Aboriginal and Torres Strait Islander people. *Cat. no. 2034.0. Canberra* 1998.

Australian Bureau of Statistics: *Deaths Australia. Cat. no. 3302.0. Canberra* 2002.

Australian Bureau of Statistics: Occasional paper: Mortality of Aboriginal and Torres Strait Islander Australians. *Cat. no. 3315.0. Canberra* 1997.

Blakely, T., Tobias, M., Robson, B., Ajwani, S., Bonne, M., Woodward, A.: Widening ethnic mortality disparities in New Zealand 1981–99. *Soc Sci Med* 2005, 61:2233–2251.

Bramley, D., Hebert, P., Jackson, R., Chassin, M.: Indigenous disparities in disease-specific mortality, a cross-country comparison: New Zealand, Australia, Canada, and the United States. *N Z Med J* 2004, 117:U1215.

Canada: Gathering Strength: Canada's Aboriginal Action Plan. Ottawa 997 [http://www.ainc-inac.gc.ca/gs/chg_e.html#reconciliation].

Canada: Report of the Royal Commission on Aboriginal Peoples. Ottawa 1996, 1–5:.

Canada: Residential Schools Settlement: Official Court Notice. Ottawa 2007 [http://www.residentialschoolsettlement.ca/english_index.html].

Cooke, M., Beavon, D., McHardy, M.: Measuring the well-being of Aboriginal People: An application of the United Nations Human Development Index to Registered Indians in Canada, 1981–2001. In Aboriginal policy research: Setting the agenda for change Volume 1. Edited by: White, J.P. Maxim, P. Beavon, D. Toronto: University of Toronto Press; 2004:47–69.

Department of Indian Affairs and Northern Development: Basic Departmental Data 2002 Ottawa: DIAND; 2003.

Department of Indian Affairs and Northern Development: Population Projections of Registered Indians, 1996–2021. Ottawa: DIAND; 1998.

Freemantle, C.J., Read, A.W., de Klerk, N.H., McAullay, D., Anderson, I.P., Stanley, F.J.: Patterns, trends, and increasing disparities in mortality for Aboriginal and non-Aboriginal infants born in Western Australia, 1980–2001: population database study. Lancet 2006, 367:1758–1766.

Hill, K., Barker, B., Vos, T.: Excess Indigenous mortality: Are Indigenous Australians more severely disadvantaged than other Indigenous populations? Int J Epidemiol 2007, 36(3):580–589.

Hunter, E., Harvey, D.: Indigenous suicide in Australia, New Zealand, Canada, and the United States. Emerg Med (Fremantle) 2002, 14:14–23.

Lavoie, J.: Governed by CONTRACTS: The development on Indigenous primary health services in Canada, Australia and New Zealand. J Abor Health 2004, 1:6–28.

Norris, M.J., Kerr, D., Nault, F.: Projections of the Population with Aboriginal Identity in Canada, 1991–2016. Report prepared by the Population Projections Section, Demography Division, Statistics Canada, for the Royal Commission on Aboriginal Peoples. Ottawa: Canada Mortgage and Housing Corporation and the Royal Commission on Aboriginal Peoples; 1995.

Olshansky, S.J., Ault, B.: The fourth stage of the epidemiologic transition: The age of delayed degenerative diseases. The Milbank Quarterly 1986, 64:355–391.

Organization for Economic Co-Operation and Development: Purchasing Power Parities Data. [http//www.oecd.org/document/47/0,2340.en_2649_34357_36202863_1_1_1_1.00.html].

Senécal, S., O'Sullivan, E.: The well-being of Inuit communities in Canada. 2006 [http://www.ainc-inac.gc.ca/pr/ra/cwb/icc/index_e.html]. Indian and Northern Affairs Canada

Statistics Canada: Life expectancy: Abridged life tables, at birth and age 65, by sex, for Canada, provinces, territories, and health regions. *CANSIM table 102-0016. Ottawa 1998.*

Statistics Canada: Life tables, Canada and provinces, 1990–92. *Cat no. 84-537. Ottawa 1995.*

Statistics New Zealand: Change in ethnicity question—2001 census of populations and dwellings. [http:www2.stats.govt.nz/domino/external/web/prod_serv. nsf/html-docChange+in+ethnicity+question+-+2001+Census+of+Populati on+and+Dwellings].

Statistics New Zealand: New Zealand life tables (1995–1997). 1999 [http:// www.stats.govt.nz/products-and.services/info-releases/nz-life-tables-info-releases.htm]. New Zealand: Statistics.

Statistics New Zealand: New Zealand life tables (2000–2002). 2004 [http:// www.stats.govt.nz/products-and-services/info-releases/nz-life-tables-info-releases.htm]. New Zealand: Statistics.

Supreme Court of Canada: R. v. Sappier; R. v. Gray. *Ottawa* 2006 [http://scc. lexum.umontreal.ca/en.2006/2006scc54/2006scc54.html].

Trovato, F.: Aboriginal mortality in Canada, the United States and New Zealand. *J Biosoc Sci* 2001, 33:67–86.

U.S. Bureau of the Census: 1990 Census of population-subject reports: education in the US. Washington: U.S. Government Printing Office; 1994.

U.S. Bureau of the Census: Census 2000 summary file 4. 2000. Report no.: SF 4

U.S. Bureau of the Census: Racial and ethnic classifications used in census 2000 and beyond. [http://www.census.gov/population/www/socdemo/race/ racefactcb.html].

ul Haq, M.: The human development paradigm. In *Readings in human development: Concepts, measures and policies for a developmental paradigm,* 2nd edition. Edited by: Fukuda-Parr, S. Shiva Kumar, A.K. New Delhi: Oxford University Press; 2005:17–34.

Verma, R., Michalowski, M., Gauvin, R.P.: Abridged life tables for registered Indians in Canada, 1976–80 to 1996–2000. *Paper presented at the annual meeting of the Population Association of America, May 1–3 2003, Minneapolis.*

CHAPTER 15

The Impact of Race and Immigrant Status on Employment Opportunities and Outcomes in Canada

Cheryl Teelucksingh and Grace-Edward Galabuzi

INTRODUCTION

The purpose of this report is to draw attention to the issue of racial discrimination in employment and its impact on the status of racialized group members in a changing Canadian labour market. We argue that the position of individuals in the Canadian labour market is determined not only by their productive capacity but also by their group affiliation and that it varies from group to group.

Labour-market attachment is critical to the livelihood and identity formation of individuals and groups, but also their ability to claim a sense of belonging and full citizenship. This is especially true of historically socially excluded groups such as racialized groups.

We present some evidence to show that in the early twenty-first-century, racial discrimination continues to deny racialized group members the attainment of their full potential in the Canadian labour market. As the data show, it is manifested in the patterns of differential access to employment, differential labour-market mobility and income inequality for racialized groups and other highly racialized groups such as recent immigrants.

CHANGES IN DEMOGRAPHICS

In the early twenty-first century, racialized groups represent a key source of human resources for the Canadian labour market. Already, 70% of net new entrants into the labour force are immigrants, 75% of whom are racialized. By 2011, 100% of net new entrants will come from this group, making the issue of racial discrimination critical to their integration into the Canadian labour market and to the success of the Canadian economy (Human Resources Development Canada, 2001). The percentage of racialized groups in the Canadian population, which was under 4% in 1971, grew to 9.4% by 1991, and reached 13.4% by 2001. In the last census period, 1996–2001, racialized group population growth outpaced that of the Canadian population, 24.6% versus 3.9%.

Racialized group population is projected to rise to 20% by 2016 partly based on its current rate of growth. Between 1996 and 2001, the working age racialized population rose by 24.6% while the racialized male proportion of the labour market grew by 28.7% and the racialized female proportion by 32.3%. According to the 2001 Census, the racialized group working age population growth was highest in Ontario (28%) and significant in British Columbia (26.6%), Alberta (22.5%), New Brunswick (18.0%), Quebec (14.7%) and only declining in Prince Edward Island (–22.6%). This compares to the general percentage change of Canada (3.9%), Ontario (6%), British Columbia (10.2%), Alberta (–1.4%), New Brunswick (–1.4%) and Quebec (1.1%).

Much of that growth can be attributed to immigration, with significant increases from Asia and the Middle East. Given Canada's continued reliance on immigration for population growth and labour-market needs, and the escalating process of globalization, these trends are likely to persist. Canada's racialized population is mainly concentrated in urban centres, with nearly three quarters (73%) living in Canada's three largest cities in 2001 and accounting for significant proportions of the populations of those municipalities—Toronto (43%), Vancouver (49%), and Montreal (23%).

In 2001, racialized group members made up 19% of the population of Ontario, Canada's largest province. That share is projected to rise to 25% by 2015. In 2001, British Columbia had the highest proportion of racialized group members in its population at 22%. While 68% of Canada's racialized group members are immigrants, a significant proportion, 32%, are Canadian-born. It is significant to note that the growth of the racialized population far outpaced that of the Canadian population in general over the last census period—1996–2001—and especially in the urban areas and the provinces of Alberta (23%), British Columbia (27%), Ontario (28%), and Quebec (15%). The size of the racialized population will continue to be an important consideration for labour market and other public policy because it is concentrated in urban Canada, which is the engine of Canada's economy.

KEY RESEARCH FINDINGS

Employment Income Attainment of Racialized and Non-racialized Groups

Income inequalities have historically been a reliable measure of racial discrimination in the labour market. The impact of racial discrimination on income distribution can be tracked using employment income data. Our analysis of that data for the period between the two census years, 1996–2001, reveals a persistent double-digit income disparity between racialized and non-racialized individual earners.

During the period, racialized group members and new immigrants experienced a median after-tax income gap of 13.3% and an average after-tax income gap of 12.2%. The gap is highest among male youth (average after-tax income gap 42.3% and median after-tax income gap 38.7%), as well as those with less than high-school education (median after-tax income gap 20.6%) and those over 65 years (average income gap 28% and median income gap 21%).

This gap is evident among the university educated (median gap 14.6%) as well as those without post-secondary education (20.6%), suggesting a cross social-class factor. But the size of the gap varies among subgroups and disappears within the family income category—likely because racialized groups have more income earners per average family.

This suggests that while the income gap between racialized and non-racialized individual earners over that period seems to be changing, it remains a significant indicator of racial inequality in the Canadian labour market.

Labour-market Participation of Racialized and Recent Immigrants

Labour-market participation rates and rates of unemployment show a continuing gap between the experience of racialized and non-racialized workers. In 2001, while the participation rates for the total population were 80.3%, those for racialized group members were as low as 66% and 75% for immigrants. Racialized groups and immigrants also experienced unequal unemployment rates, with the total population rate being 6.7% while the racialized group rate was as high as 12.6%.

Sectoral Distribution for Racialized and Non-racialized Groups

The labour market is segmented along racial lines, with racialized group members overrepresented in many low-paying occupations with high levels of precariousness while they are under-represented in the better-paying, more secure jobs. Racialized groups were overrepresented in textile, light manufacturing and service sector occupations such as sewing machine operators (46%), electronic assemblers (42%), plastics processing (36.8%), labourers in textile processing (40%), taxi and limo drivers (36.6%), weavers and knitters (37.5%), fabrics, fur and leather cutters (40.1%), and ironing and pressing (40.6%).

They were under-represented in senior management (8.2%), professionals (13.8%), supervisors (12%), fire-fighters (2.0%), legislators (2.2%), oil and gas drilling (1.5%), and farmers and farm managers (1.2%). One area where they fared better is in the information technology industry, with software engineers (36.3%), computer engineers (30.1%), and computer programmers (27.8%).

Converting Human Capital Investment into Occupational Status and Compensation

Yet another key indicator of racial inequality is the ability of racialized group members to translate their investment in human capital in terms of educational attainment into comparable occupational status and compensation. The shift towards more immigrants from the South has led to a noticeable lag in economic attainment among members of the immigrant groups. This has occurred despite the 1990s emphasis on skilled immigrants in immigration policy. Ironically, as the selection process has become more stringent in response to charges that immigrant quality has declined, a majority of immigrants from the

South now come through the independent (skilled) class—over 60% in recent years (Citizenship & Immigration Canada, 2001).

For many racialized group members, educational attainment has not translated into comparable labour-market access, or workplace mobility. In 2001, racialized group members were overrepresented among highly educated categories such as holders of bachelor's, master's, and doctorate degrees. However, they were under-represented under the trade and college graduate ranks, as well as among those with less than a grade 12–13 education. According to a Conference Board of Canada study (2004), while racialized groups averaged less than 11% of the labour force between 1992 and 2000, they accounted for 0.3% of real gross domestic product (GDP) growth. That contrasts with the remaining 89% of the labour force that contributed 0.6%. This disproportionately larger contribution to GDP growth is likely to grow over the 2002–2016 period as the contribution of the rest of the population falls. However, this productivity was not rewarded, as the average wages for racialized groups over that period remained 14.5% lower than that of other Canadians. The Board report concludes that in monetary terms, over the period 1992 to 2016, racialized groups will contribute $80.9 billion in real GDP growth.

Differential Access to Professions and Trades

In the early twenty-first century, an important aspect of the experience of racialized groups in the Canadian labour market is the experience of those whose education is obtained abroad. This category, here referred to as internationally educated professionals and trades people (IEPs), has been growing as Canada's immigration system has moved towards more stringent selection criteria, with emphasis on higher education and market-oriented skills. In the first three years of the new millennium, over 60% of newcomers had university degrees.

Because of their increasingly significant numbers as a proportion of the racialized cohort, their experience, while specific, in part explains the failure of racialized group members to translate their educational attainment and experience into higher occupational status, intra- and inter-sectoral mobility and compensation.

It also speaks directly to the failure of the major players—governments, licensing bodies and other regulators, employers, educational institutions, trade unions (and perhaps the IEPs themselves) to devise appropriate policy and program responses to the problem of inequitable access to professions and trades and to ensure a smooth transition for internationally trained professionals and tradespeople into their fields of expertise.

A successful integration strategy would require a focus on evaluating the competencies of trained immigrants rather than on demands for undefined Canadian experience, approximating the value of their human capital based on what source country they are from and proposing to send them without supports to non-urban environments as a condition of their residence. It would mean state-supported efforts to match immigrant skills with the labour-market shortages that exist in Canada's regions, provinces and cities, towns, and communities. The Canadian government has a history of supporting past immigration with such resources as land for settlement. In this case, however, it has embarked on the selection of highly talented immigrants but assumed no accountability for their successful integration or even bothered to track their progress. Instead, even as it pursues a laissez-faire approach to their integration, it continues to compete for immigrants bearing similar skills, raising troubling questions about the logic of this aggressive immigration policy.

Surprisingly, in the case of the debate on the brain drain to the USA, the federal and provincial governments have responded by implementing taxation and other policy measures aimed at discouraging skilled immigration to the United States. However, despite demands for similar action by IEPs, communities and increasingly employers, equitable access to professions and trades in Canada has remained on the policy back burner. Ironically, in terms of sheer numbers, Canada receives four skilled immigrants for every one that migrates to the USA. Moreover, they are as or even more highly skilled than the ones leaving (Canada attracts more master's and doctoral graduates than it loses), and have chosen to live and work in Canada. Yet the issue of the brain waste has not prompted policy action adequate to the problem.

THE NATURE OF THE PROBLEM

Internationally educated immigrants are supposed to be the future of Canada's increasingly labour-strapped economy. With massive baby boom retirements on the horizon, someone has to pay their pensions and keep the tax dollars flowing for the social programs they will need in their old age.

Canada also promises the IEPs an opportunity to improve their lives and those of their families. It seems like a win–win proposition. This proposition, however, depends on the relatively seamless integration of IEPs into their fields of expertise. Yet, not unlike their predecessors, this group of largely racialized immigrants confronts a Canadian labour market with racial hierarchies, with structures of discrimination that defy the logic articulated above.

With governments in a neo-liberal era committed to deregulating the labour market rather than intervening in failed labour markets to ensure the optimal allocation of human resources, IEPs are impacted by the full weight of subjective decision-making on the part of employers. The racial composition of the immigration group began to change in the 1960s, and by the 1980s that process was in full stride. It seemed to coincide with a period during which the state and self-regulating professional and occupational bodies imposed strict administration of rules and regulations in the name of ensuring the public interest, a process that has had the effect of erecting new barriers to entry for many recently immigrated IEPs. While the labour-market conditions that precipitated the defensive actions have changed, the regulators have been slow to respond to the growing demands for licensing newcomers.

Furthermore, not all occupations or trades are regulated, and some are more regulated than others, which leads to varied experiences and leaves decisions at the behest of employers.

Employers' attitudes towards internationally obtained skills and their bearers have been identified as particularly problematic. There is some general agreement around some of the issues that need to be addressed:

- Lack of adequate information about the licensing process, pre- and post-arrival
- Paucity of reliable tools for assessing credentials and other prior learning
- Lack of competency-based licensing and sector-specific language testing
- Inadequate bridging and supplementary training and internship opportunities
- Limited transparency in the licensing process and lack of feedback or an appeal process
- Limited co-ordination between stakeholders

POLICY RESPONSES

Most of the issues identified herein are within the purview of public policy and can be addressed by governments in partnership with regulators, educational institutions, assessment agencies, trade unions, employers, and service providers.

There is a need to define the public interest as including a focus on equity and economic efficiency. This need has never been greater than it is in this globalized labour-market environment. The systemic failure to properly evaluate and accredit prior learning by employers and regulators casts them not as defenders of the public interest but as gatekeepers and lacking transparency in the application processes.

Along with the existence of closed trade union shops, these factors make it difficult to review their excise of discretion to eliminate the barriers. The effect is the devaluation and degrading of the skills of vulnerable IEPs, which contributes to documented occupational and wage inequality. Although IEPs, immigrants and racialized communities are organizing to challenge this exercise of power, they are often powerless to stop their victimization and require governments to take the responsibility of enforcing a broader definition of the public interest.

CONCLUSION

While far outpacing the general Canadian population growth, and contributing a majority of new entrants into the labour market, racialized groups and immigrants have not fared well in the labour market in the last census period (1996–2001).

A review of employment income data and labour-market participation patterns of racialized groups and recent immigrants during the last census period (1996–2001) shows both a double-digit income gap between racialized and non-racialized populations in the Canadian labour market, higher unemployment and lower participation rates, and concentrations in the low-income occupations.

These patterns are evident even when educational attainment is taken into account, suggesting that racialized group members and recent immigrants are not able to translate their educational attainment (indeed advantage) into comparable occupational status and compensation. This is partly explained by the experience of internationally educated professionals who face barriers to converting their skills into skilled occupations. There are variations in the size of the gap among subgroups and it seems to disappear when you consider family income—with racialized groups having more income earners per family. There is a noticeable gap between racialized men and women, suggesting a gendered dimension to the inequality identified. This analysis is confirmed by the findings from interviews with key informants from among settlement sector officials in Vancouver, Calgary, Toronto, Montreal, and Halifax, where over 80% of the racialized and recent immigrant population lives. Read together with the unequal unemployment rates, the inability of racialized group members to convert their educational attainment advantage into commensurate occupational status and income, the differential experiences of internationally trained racialized group members and the sectoral concentrations, the findings confirm the racialized groups' experience of racial inequality in the Canadian labour market and the persistence of racial discrimination in employment.

The impact of racial discrimination in employment in the early twenty-first century is amplified because of the size of the racialized population, but also because the population's contribution to the Canadian economy has grown exponentially over the last two decades. The stakes are high because race continues to be a major factor in the distribution of opportunities in the Canadian labour market and by extension in determining the life chances of racialized peoples and immigrants in Canada. The major difference is that this disadvantage will now translate into a drag on the Canadian economy and the Canadian population as a whole.

REFERENCES

Brouwer, A. *Immigrants Need Not Apply*. Ottawa: Caledon Institute of Social Policy, 1999.

Citizenship and Immigration Canada. *Facts and Figures 2001*. Ottawa: Government of Canada, 2001.

Conference Board of Canada. *Making a Visible Difference: The Contributions of Visible Minorities to Canadian Economic Growth*. Ottawa: Conference Board of Canada, 2004.

Li, P. *Destination Canada: Immigration Debates and Issues.* Toronto: Wall & Thompson, 2003.

Reitz, J.G. "Immigrant Skill Utilization in the Canadian Labour Market: Implications of Human Capital Research." *Journal of International Migration and Integration* 2, no. 3 (Summer 2001): 347–378.

FURTHER READING

Abbott, C. and C. Beach, "Immigrant Earnings Differentials and Birth-Year Effects of Men in Canada: Post-War–1972." *Canadian Journal of Economics* 26 August 1993, 505–524.

Abella, R. *Equality Now: Report of the Commission on Equality in Employment.* Ottawa: Supply and Services Canada, 1984.

Akbari, A. *The Economics of Immigration and Racial Discrimination: A Literature Survey (1970-1989).* Ottawa: Multiculturalism & Citizenship Canada, 1989.

——. "Immigrant 'Quality' in Canada: More Direct Evidence of Human Capital Content, 1956–1994." *International Migration Review* 33 (Spring 1999): 156–175.

Alboim, N., R. Finnie and M. Skuterud. *Immigrants' Skills in the Canadian Labour market: Empirical Evidence and Policy Issues.* Mimeo, 2003.

Anisef, P., R. Sweeet and G. Frempong. *Labour Market Outcomes of Immigrant and Racial Minority University Graduates in Canada.* CERIS working paper No. 23. CERIS, March 2003.

Arrow, K. "What Has Economics to Say about Racial Discrimination?" *Journal of Economic Perspectives* 12, no. 2 (Spring 1998): 91–100.

Bakan, A., and A. Kobayashi. *Employment Equity Policy in Canada: An Interprovincial Comparison.* Ottawa: Status of Women Canada, 2000.

Baker, M. and D. Benjamin. "The Performance of Immigrants in the Canadian Labour Market." *Journal of Labour Economics* 12 (1994): 369–405.

Basran, G.S. and L. Zong "Devaluation of Foreign Credentials as Perceived by Visible Minority Professional Immigrants." *Canadian Ethnic Studies* 30, no. 3 (1998): 6–23.

Beach, C. and C. Worswick, "Is there a Double-Negative Effect on the Earnings of Immigrant Women?" *Canadian Public Policy* 19, no. 1 (1993): 36–53.

Bloom, M. and M. Grant. *Brain Gain: The Economic Benefits of Recognizing Learning Credentials in Canada.* Ottawa: Conference Board of Canada, 2001.

Boyd, M. "Gender, Visible Minority and Immigrant Earnings Inequality: Reassessing and Employment Equity Premise." In *Deconstructing a Nation: Immigration, Multiculturalism and Racism in the 1990s Canada*, ed. V. Satzewich. Toronto: Garamond Press, 1992.

Calleja, D. "Right Skills, Wrong Country." *Canadian Business*, 26 June 2000, www. skillsforchange.org/news/other/canadian_business_news_june_2000. htm.

Canadian Human Rights Commission. *Employment Equity Annual Reports*, 1996–1999.

Citizenship and Immigration Canada. *The Economic Performance of Immigrants: Immigration Category Perspective, 1998.* Ottawa: Government of Canada, 2000.

——. *The Economic Performance of Immigrants: Education Perspective, Strategic policy, Planning and Research.* Ottawa: Government of Canada, 2000.

——. *Skilled Worker Immigrants: Towards a New Model of Selection.* Ottawa: Government of Canada, 1998.

De Voretz, D.J., ed.. *Diminishing Returns: the Economics of Canada's Recent Immigration Policy.* Toronto: C.D. Howe Institute, 1995.

Fernando, T. and K. Prasad. *Multiculturalism and Employment Equity: Problems Facing Foreign-Trained Professionals and Trades People in British Columbia.* Vancouver: Affiliation of Multicultural Societies and Services of British Columbia, 1986.

Frenette, M. and R. Morissette. *Will they ever converge? Earnings of immigrants and Canadian-born workers over the last two decades.* Analytical Studies paper No. 215. Ottawa: Statistics Canada, 2003.

Galabuzi, G. *Canada's Creeping Economic Apartheid: The Economic Segregation and Social Marginalization of Racialized Groups.* Toronto: CJS Foundation for Research & Education, 2001.

Grant, H. and R. Oertel. "Diminishing Returns to Immigration? Interpreting the Economic Experience of Canadian Immigrants." *Canadian Ethnic Studies* 30, no. 3 (1998): 57–76.

Harvey, E.B. and B. Siu. "Immigrants' Socioeconomic Situation Compared, 1991–1996." *INSCAN* 15, No. 2 (Fall 2001): 1–3.

Henry, F. and E. Ginsberg. *Who Gets the Job: A Test of Racial Discrimination in Employment.* Toronto: Urban Alliance on Race Relations/Social Planning Council of Metro Toronto, 1985.

Hou, F. and T. Balakrishnan, "The Integration of Visible Minorities in Contemporary Canadian Society." *Canadian Journal of Sociology* 21, no. 3 (1996): 307–326.

House of Commons. *Equality Now! Report of the Special Committee on the Participation of Visible Minorities in Canadian Society.* Ottawa: Government of Canada, 1984.

Human Resources Development Canada. "Recent Immigrants Have Experienced Unusual Economic Difficulties." *Applied Research Bulletin* 7, no. 1 (Winter/ Spring, 2001).

Jackson, A. *Is Work Working for Workers of Colour?* Ottawa: Canadian Labour Congress, 2002.

Jain, H. *Employment Discrimination Against Visible Minorities and Employment Equity.* Hamilton: McMaster University, 1988.

Li, P. *Ethnic Inequality in a Class Society.* Toronto: Wall & Thompson, 1988.

——. "The Market Worth of Immigrants' Educational Credential." *Canadian Public Policy* 27, no. 1 (2001): 23–38.

Lundahl, M. and E. Wadensjo. *Unequal Treatment: A Study in the Neo-classical Theory of Discrimination.* New York: New York University Press, 1984.

Mata, F. "The Non-Accreditation of Immigrant Professionals in Canada: Societal Impacts, Barriers and Present Policy Initiatives." Paper presented at Sociology and Anthropology Meetings, University of Calgary, 3 June 1994.

Ontario Ministry of Training, Colleges and Universities. *The Facts Are In: A Study of the Characteristics and Experiences of Immigrants Seeking Employment in Regulated Professions in Ontario.* Toronto: Queen's Printer, 2002.

Pendukar, K. and R. Pendukar. "The Colour of Money: Earnings Differentials among Ethnic Groups in Canada." *Canadian Journal of Economics* 31, no. 3 (1998): 518–548.

Reitz, J.G. "Immigrant Skill Utilization in the Canadian Labour Market: Implications of Human Capital Research." *Journal of International Migration and Integration* 2, no. 3 (Summer 2001): 347–378.

Sangster, D. *Assessing and Recognizing Foreign Credentials in Canada: Employers' Views.* Ottawa: Canadian Labour and Business Centre, 2001.

Siddiqui, H. "Immigrants Subsidize Us by $55 Billion per Year." *Toronto Star,* 14 January 2001.

Stasiulis, D. "Affirmative Action for Visible Minorities and the New Politics of Race in Canada." In *Canada 2000 Race Relations and Public Policy,* ed. O.P. Dwivedi et al. Guelph: University of Guelph, 1989.

Stoffman, D. *Towards a More Realistic Immigration Policy for Canada.* Toronto: C.D. Howe Institute, 1993.

CHAPTER 16

Employment and Persons with Disabilities in Canada

Canadian Council on Social Development

In this 18th edition of the CCSD's *Disability Research Information Sheets*, we provide various employment-related statistics for persons with disabilities in Canada, using data from the 2001 Participation and Activity Limitation Survey (PALS),[1] the 2001 Workplace and Employee Survey (WES),[2] and the 2001 Census of the Population.[3] We also provide a brief summary of some of the findings of a report entitled *Supports and Services for Adults and Children Aged 5–14 with Disabilities in Canada* and, in particular, the requirements and unmet needs for employment supports and services. This longer report was commissioned by the Federal-Provincial-Territorial Ministers Responsible for Social Services and released on December 3, 2004. (www.socialunion. ca/pwd_e.html)

EMPLOYMENT SUPPORTS

Modified Work Structures

Among *employed* persons with disabilities, 15% report that they need some type of "modified work structure" in or around the workplace. This would include structures such as handrails/ramps; accessible parking; accessible elevators; modified workstations; accessible washrooms; accessible transportation; and "other" structures. The most commonly required work structure is a modified workstation (required by 7%), followed by accessible parking (5%).[4] (Note: some individuals require modifications to more than one structure.)

The rate of requirement for modified work structures in or around the workplace is even higher among persons with disabilities who are *unemployed*. In fact, unemployed workers with disabilities are nearly twice as likely (28%) as those who are employed to require some type of modified work structure.[5] It may be that this requirement for modified workplace structures leaves an individual more vulnerable to job loss or to greater difficulty in finding employment.

Work Aids or Job Modifications

In addition to modifications to work structures—which may be thought of as infrastructure changes—some individuals have requirements for more personal or individualized supports, which are referred to as "work aids or job modifications." These would include: job redesign (modified or different duties); modified work hours; human supports (such as readers, sign-language interpreters, job coaches, personal assistants); technical aids (such as a voice synthesizer, TTY or TDD, infrared system, portable note-takers); a computer with Braille, large print, speech access, or a scanner; communication aids (such as Braille or large-print reading material or recording equipment); and "other."

Employed persons with disabilities are more likely to require work aids or job modifications than they are to require modified work structures. About 30% of employed persons with disabilities require some type of work aid or job modification, with modified work hours (required by 19% of employed persons with disabilities) and job redesign (required by 17%) being the most commonly cited.[6]

Among *unemployed* persons with disabilities, 56% say they require some type of work aid or job modification, with job redesign (required by 42%) and modified work hours (35%) being the most commonly cited.[7] This suggests that a requirement for work aids or job modifications may be linked to job instability. (Note: some individuals require more than one type of aid or modification.)

Unmet Needs

Among *employed* persons with disabilities, the greatest rate of unmet need for modified work structures is accessible transportation—26% of those who require it, don't have it. Roughly one in five who require handrails/ramps, accessible parking, accessible elevators, or accessible workstations have an unmet need, and 12% who require accessible washrooms have an unmet need. In terms of sheer numbers, the greatest unmet need is for modified workstations (an unmet need for 10,900 persons) and for accessible parking (an unmet need for 8,140 persons).

Among this group, the greatest *rate* of unmet need for work aids or job modifications is for "other" (unspecified) work aids (29% with this unmet need) and for technical aids (27% unmet need). In terms of *numbers*, the greatest unmet need is for modified work hours (unmet need for 152,280) and job redesign (unmet need for 138,190).

Why is Workplace Accommodation so Problematic?

Our findings from the 2001 PALS indicate that there is a fairly high requirement for some type of workplace accommodation among those with disabilities, but these requirements are often for things that do not seem difficult to provide. Since modified workstations and accessible parking are the most commonly required structures, and modified work hours and job redesign are the most commonly required aids, one might think that these items would be relatively simple to provide. Instead, however, a fairly high number of individuals have unmet needs for these items, and these unmet needs can act as major barriers to their labour-force participation and economic security.

In a recent report by the Canadian Abilities Foundation (CAF) using data gathered specifically for their study, similar conclusions are drawn. While the requirement for workplace accommodations is fairly high,[8] these accommodations are usually not terribly costly. They estimated that "annual workplace accommodation costs are under $1,500 for almost all workers who have a disability."[9] According to their study, for just over half of those requiring some type of accommodation, the estimated cost would be less than $500 per person per year; for one-third, the cost would be $500 to $1,500 per year; and for 16%, the cost was estimated at over $1,500. These costs are probably much lower than many employers realize. For many persons with disabilities, an employer's reluctance to provide accommodation on the job can be extremely disheartening and frustrating: "Employers are still ignorant about what it takes to hire and accommodate a person with a disability."[10]

Despite our findings that workers with disabilities often require some flexibility in the workplace, there is evidence that they may actually face *less* flexibility than do workers without disabilities. In the CAF report, strategies such as "flexible work hours" and "working at home" are cited as methods of accommodating many workers with disabilities. However, using data from the 2001 WES, we find that workers without disabilities are more likely than those with disabilities to be able to work from home (23.6%, compared to 15.9%). Workers without disabilities are also more likely to report having flexible work hours (35.5% compared to 29.5% for workers with disabilities).

These differences may be related to the kinds of jobs or types of employers that the workers have, or they may be related to differences in the manner in which workers with and without disabilities are treated. Certainly, these findings suggest that there may be room for greater flexibility for workers with disabilities.

There are also some interesting findings coming out of the United States. Since 1984, the US Department of Labor, Office of Disability Employment Policy, has provided a toll-free service known as the Job Accommodation Network (JAN). JAN provides advice regarding workplace accommodations to persons with disabilities and to employers. In a one-year period between October 1994 and September 1995, JAN received over 80,000 calls. Of the businesses seeking advice on workplace accommodation, the solution for 19% had no cost attached; for another 50%, the cost of accommodation was between $1 and $500. Only 3% reported a cost of more than $5,000. Even more interesting is the fact that the majority of these businesses also reported receiving some type of financial return as a result of implementing the workplace accommodation. In fact, the average return was $28.69 for every $1 spent on accommodation.

LABOUR FORCE INSTABILITY

According to the 2001 PALS, just under one-quarter (22.3%) of employed persons with disabilities reported having had at least one period of unemployment in the previous year. There was only a slight variation by gender—with women at 23.1% and men at

21.6%—and by level of education.[11] However, both the worker's age and severity of disability appear to leave persons with disabilities more vulnerable to unemployment. For example, 27.7% of workers with severe or very severe disabilities faced unemployment within the previous year, compared with 22.2% among those with moderate disabilities, and 19.7% of those with mild disabilities (Figure 16.1).

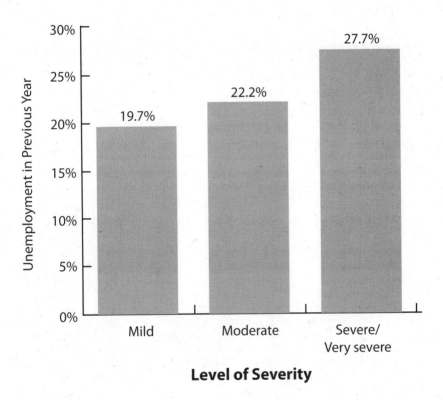

Figure 16.1: Workers with Disabilities Who Experienced Unemployment in the Previous Year, by Severity of Disability

Source: Calculations by the CCSD using data from Statistics Canada's Participation and Activity Limitation Survey (PALS), 2001.

As well, younger workers with disabilities are more likely than their older counterparts to face unemployment. As seen in Figure 16.2, 30.5% of workers aged 15 to 34 with disabilities faced unemployment within the previous year, compared with 20.6% of those aged 35 to 44, and 19.9% of those aged 45 to 64. As documented here and in other studies, younger workers with disabilities tend to face higher levels of disadvantage in the labour market in a number of areas, and facing this type of disadvantage early in life can have a cumulative negative impact on one's career possibilities.

For 13% of workers with disabilities, their employment is not permanent in nature.[12] There is only a slight variation by level of severity and by gender, but age is an important factor: 19.8% of those aged 15 to 34 worked at a non-permanent job, compared with 10.1% of those aged 45 to 64 (Figure 16.3).[13]

Figure 16.3: Workers with Disabilities in Non-permanent Jobs, by Age Group

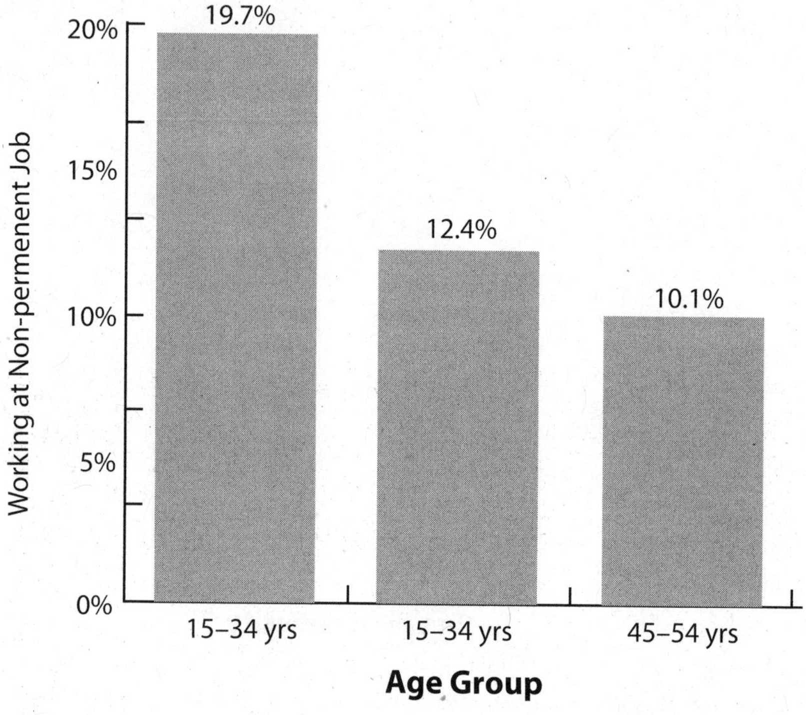

Source: Calculations by the CCSD using data from Statistics Canada's Participation and Activity Limitation Survey (PALS), 2001.

LABOUR-MARKET ACTIVITY

Using data from the 2001 Census, we examined labour force activity over a one-year period for the working-age population (aged 15 to 64 years). At the national level, it is clear that adults with disabilities are considerably less likely than their non-disabled counterparts to have a full-time, full-year work profile. They are also much more likely to have had no activity in the paid labour force at all.

Men without disabilities are the most likely to have been employed full-time for the full year, and women with disabilities are the least likely to have this profile. For example, 53.2% of men without disabilities had full-time, full-year employment in 2000, compared with 34.9% of men with disabilities, 37.4% of women without disabilities, and 23.2% of women with disabilities (Table 16.1).[14] Similarly, 12.8% of men without disabilities did not work at all in 2000, compared with 36.5% of men with disabilities, 22.5% of women without disabilities, and 46.7% of women with disabilities.

This general relationship held true within every province and territory, although it was more pronounced in some than in others. Table 16.2 summarizes the percentage of men and women, with and without disabilities, who worked full-time for the full year in 2000, by province and territory.

Table 16.1: Work Activity for Women and Men with and without Disabilities, 2000

	Worked 49 to 52 weeks		Worked less than 49 weeks		
	Full-time, full-year	Part-time, full-year	Full-time, part-year	Part-time, part-year	Did not work during year
Women with disabilities	23.2%	6.7%	12.5%	11.0%	46.7%
Men with disabilities	34.9%	2.9%	18.4%	7.2%	36.5%
Women without disabilities	37.4%	9.1%	17.0%	14.1%	22.5%
Men without disabilities	53.2%	3.5%	22.2%	8.3%	12.8%

Source: Calculations by the CCSD using data from Statistics Canada's Census, 2001.

Figure 16.2: Workers with Disabilities who Experienced Unemployment in the Previous Year, by Age Group

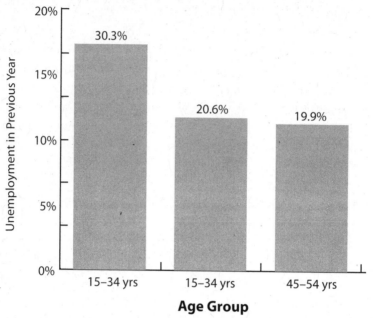

Source: Calculations by the CCSD using data from Statistics Canada's Participation and Activity Limitation Survey (PALS), 2001.

Table 16.2: Percent of Persons,* with and without Disabilities, Who Worked Full-time Full-year in 2000, by Gender and Province/Territory

	With Disabilities		Without Disabilities	
	Women	**Men**	**Women**	**Men**
CAN.	23.2%	34.9%	37.4%	53.2%
NFLD & LB	15.0%	17.1%	28.1%	34.7%
PEI	22.4%	30.1%	36.0%	44.7%
NS	18.6%	28.9%	34.9%	49.3%
NB	19.0%	28.1%	35.2%	46.7%
QC	16.6%	24.8%	35.3%	50.1%
ON	24.8%	38.3%	40.3%	57.2%
MB	28.3%	41.2%	40.6%	57.3%
SK	27.6%	41.0%	38.2%	53.9%
AB	28.2%	43.3%	38.6%	57.0%
BC	22.6%	33.5%	33.4%	48.4%
YK	34.5%	34.3%	41.9%	44.8%
NWT	33.8%	42.1%	42.6%	50.2%
NU	19.8%	27.0%	28.2%	36.3%

*Persons aged 15 to 64.
Source: Calculated by the CCSD using data from Statistics Canada's 2001 Census.

It is in the territories that the percentages of full-time, full-year work are most alike among adults with and without disabilities. In the Northwest Territories, for example, the rate of working full-time, full-year for men without disabilities is 1.2 times that of men with disabilities; for women, the corresponding figure is 1.3 times. There are similar relationships in the Yukon and in Nunavut, although in Nunavut the rate of full-time, full-year work is low for all groups. Rates of full-time, full-year work among those with and those without disabilities were least alike in Quebec and in Newfoundland and Labrador. In those two provinces, adults without disabilities were about twice as likely as those with disabilities to have worked full-time for the full year.

In every province and territory in 2000, persons with disabilities were more likely than those without disabilities to have had no employment during the year (Table 16.3). Here again, the gap varied somewhat by geography. Among men in Prince Edward Island, for example, the percentage of those with disabilities who were without employment for the full year was nearly four times (3.89) that of men without disabilities (31% compared with 8%). And in New Brunswick, Nova Scotia, Quebec, and Ontario, the percentage of men with disabilities who were without work for the year was over three times that of their non-disabled counterparts. The gap was smallest in Nunavut. Among women, the gap between those with and those without disabilities was smaller than it was among men. Like men, however, the differences were greatest in Prince Edward Island and smallest in Nunavut.

Table 16.3: Percent of Persons,* with and without Disabilities, Who Did Not Work During the Year 2000, by Gender and Province/Territory

	With Disabilities		Without Disabilities	
	Women	Men	Women	Men
CAN.	46.7%	36.5%	22.5%	12.8%
NFLD & LB	61.0%	55.1%	32.3%	19.1%
PEI	38.8%	31.0%	14.4%	8.0%
NS	53.6%	44.4%	24.3%	13.4%
NB	51.4%	42.4%	22.8%	12.5%
QC	59.3%	49.6%	27.0%	15.7%
ON	46.1%	35.3%	20.6%	11.5%
MB	39.2%	29.4%	18.9%	10.7%
SK	36.9%	28.3%	18.9%	11.7%
AB	35.6%	23.7%	17.5%	8.3%
BC	43.1%	33.4%	23.1%	14.2%
YK	21.5%	18.5%	11.9%	8.5%
NWT	29.7%	22.1%	17.0%	11.2%
NU	42.2%	29.0%	29.2%	21.5%

*Persons aged 15 to 64.

Source: Calculated by the CCSD using data from Statistics Canada's 2001 Census.

ENDNOTES

1. The Adult PALS is a post-censal survey, that is, a survey that uses a Census question to identify the target population. It was conducted in 10 provinces and contains rich disability-specific information, such as severity rate and type of disability.

2. The 2001 WES surveyed employed individuals and their employers. Excluded from this survey were workplaces involved in: public administration; crop and animal production; fishing, hunting, and trapping; private households; religious organizations; and workplaces in the Territories. Because public administration was excluded, there is a heavy emphasis on private sector employers. The 2001 WES surveyed over 20,000 employees in more than 5,000 workplaces.

3. Screening questions concerning "activity limitations" are contained in the Census Long Form, which was distributed to one in five Canadians.

4. Among employed persons with disabilities, rates of requirement for other structures are as follows: accessible elevators (4%); accessible washrooms (4%); accessible transportation (3%); handrails/ramps (3%); and "other" (1%).

5. Among unemployed persons with disabilities, rates of requirement for specific structures are as follows: accessible parking (12%); modified workstations (12%); accessible elevators (10%); accessible washrooms (8%); accessible transportation (8%); handrails/ramps (6%); and "other" (1%).

6. Among employed persons with disabilities, rates of requirement for other specific work aids or job modifications are: "other" (5%); human supports (3%); technical aids (2%); and computer with Braille (1%).

7. Among unemployed persons with disabilities, rates of requirement for other specific work aids or job modifications are: human supports (10%); "other" (6%); and technical aids (4%).

8. In this study, the rate of requirement is higher than was found in our study. However, in the CAF study, the population surveyed included both those who were working and those who were not working (some of whom were not actively looking for work but had worked within the last five years). This difference would tend to increase the proportion of those who might have a requirement.

9. Canadian Abilities Foundation. *Neglected or Hidden*. Toronto: CAF, 2004, p. 9.

10. *Ibid.*

11. Less than high school, 23.6%; high school graduate, 22.7%; and post-secondary graduate, 21.7%.

12. Non-permanent jobs include seasonal work, contract or term work, casual jobs, work done through a temporary help agency, and the like.

13. Among those aged 35 to 44, 12.4% were in non-permanent jobs.

14. More investigation using age breakdowns needs to be done on these data in the future. Persons with disabilities tend, on average, to be older than those without disabilities. Part—but certainly not all—of these differences are likely due to early retirement of a higher proportion of persons with disabilities. However, even if we consider that, due to differences in the age distribution of the two populations, persons with disabilities may be less likely to have been employed because they were retired, we must remember that a certain proportion of that retirement may not be entirely voluntary. It is likely that many individuals retire from the labour market due to disability.

CHAPTER 17

A Call to Combat Poverty and Exclusion of Canadians with Disabilities

Council of Canadians with Disabilities

The Council of Canadians with Disabilities (CCD) and the Canadian Association for Community Living (CACL) are calling on the federal government to take principled and committed leadership in Budget 2005 to combat the poverty and exclusion of Canadians with disabilities. There is now an unprecedented consensus among the Canadian public, governments, the disability community and experts about the need for national action on disability, in particular to ensure access to needed supports.

Prime Minister Martin

> *"What kind of Canada do we want? ... a Canada where people with disabilities and their families ... have the support they need."*
>
> Response to the Speech from the Throne, February 2004

The Canadian Public

> *"More than eight in ten [Canadians] ... agree with the statement that persons with even the most challenging disabilities should be supported by public funds to live in the community rather than institutional settings ... By a wide margin, Canadians believe governments have the primary role for supporting persons with disabilities when it comes to providing good health care, reliable transportation, specialized equipment, and good education."*
>
> From Environics, "Canadian Attitudes Towards Disability Issues," 2004

BACKGROUND TO THE ISSUE

With the aging of the population, people with disabilities make up a growing proportion of the Canadian population. One third of Aboriginal Canadians are disabled. Canadians with disabilities are more than twice as likely to live in poverty than other Canadians. They face exclusion from quality education, from employment and from participation in their communities. Rates of violence and abuse against people with disabilities are among the highest for any group in Canadian society.

Current investments by governments are not making the difference needed. Recent analysis commissioned by the Federal and Provincial/Territorial Ministers Responsible for Social Services dramatically illustrates how this group of Canadians is still marked by poverty and exclusion.[1]

The first step in combating poverty and exclusion is to ensure people have access to the disability-related supports they need: aids and devices, personal assistance, environmental accommodations, etc. With the right supports—that are flexible and responsive as people age and make transitions to new life stages—people with disabilities learn, become employed, raise families, and contribute to their communities and to the social and economic well-being of Canada.

Adults with disabilities, when they get the supports they need, establish their independence from their parental families and often become caregivers of their own children. Access to needed supports is the central foundation for inclusion and equal participation of Canadians with disabilities.[2]

Yet as recent reports indicate, a significant number of children, youth, and adults with disabilities lack the supports they need because they are too costly or aren't available where they live, or because schools, workplaces, transportation systems, and public spaces are not designed to include them. Drawing on Statistics Canada data, The Roeher Institute estimates that nearly two thirds of Canadian adults with disabilities—2,154,000 people—face one or more such difficulties.

> Over two million Canadians adults with disabilities, or two thirds of the disabled adult population, lack one or more of the educational, workplace, aids, home modification, or other supports they need.

Roeher estimates that the non-reimbursed costs to individuals of purchasing their needed disability supports is about $4.2 billion per annum.[3] And many have such needs but don't have the income to purchase the required supports.

Public policy has not yet caught up with the social, economic, and demographic realities of disability in Canada nor has it provided the foundations to ensure the full inclusion of Canadians with disabilities and a quality of life equal to other Canadians.

Speech from the Throne, October 2004
> *"The Government's actions on behalf of Canadians will be guided by [a] commitment to defend the Charter of Rights and Freedoms and to be a steadfast advocate of inclusion."*

THE TIME FOR ACTION IS NOW

Recognizing the need for a new approach, the federal and provincial/territorial governments signed the In Unison Accord[4] in 1998 to advance the full citizenship, inclusion, and participation of Canadians with disabilities. It identifies access to *disability supports* as a critical building block to enable better income and employment status for Canadians with disabilities. As of yet, however, a National Framework to put In Unison into action has not been established.

The Standing Committee on Finance
> *"The federal government [should] meet with provincial/territorial governments and groups representing the disabled with a view to concluding a federal/provincial/territorial national disability strategy ... Moreover, the government should review and implement, on an expeditious basis, the recommendations of the Technical Advisory Committee on Tax Measures for Persons with Disabilities."*
> From "Moving Forward: Balancing Priorities and Making Choices for the Economy of the Twenty-First Century," Report of the Standing Committee, December 2004.

Based on various consultations with other disability organizations, experts and governments, CCD and CACL have developed the following recommendations for a National Framework and Agenda.

SHORT-TERM STRATEGIES—1–2 YEARS

In the 2005 Budget, the Federal Government should:

1. **Commit to a Framework for Investment in Disability Supports**—The framework would be based on the vision and principles of In Unison; will be

developed in collaboration with provincial and territorial governments and First Nations; and will assist individuals to meet the costs of disability-related supports, support family/informal caregivers, and enable community capacity to provide supports and inclusion.

2. **Implement recommendations to Ministers of Finance and Revenue in Disability Tax Fairness**—Move quickly to implement the Report's recommendations. The cost of these recommendations was booked in previous federal budgets.

3. **Make a "down payment" on a transfer to enhance the supply of disability supports, and commit to a national program starting 2006**—Make a down payment in Budget 2005 for a transfer to provinces and territories to enhance disability supports using the "Multilateral Framework for Labour Market Agreements for Persons with Disabilities" as a model for wider investments in disability supports. Commit to an investment in disability supports beginning in 2006 significant enough to make a national program a reality (possibly using a renegotiated Multi-Lateral Framework Agreement).

4. **Commit to a "disability dimension" in new initiatives, including Caregivers, Childcare, Cities and Communities, and the Gas Tax Rebate**—The federal government has already committed to a principle of "universal inclusion" in its childcare strategy. Similar commitments should be made in infrastructure initiatives for cities and communities, including the Gas Tax Rebate, to enhance accessible transportation and other services.

5. **Commit to a study of poverty and disability**—As a foundation for exploring an expanded role for the federal government in addressing income needs.

6. **Engage the disability community and provincial/territorial governments in developing the agenda**—By resourcing the disability community to effectively engage, and by establishing a new high level Technical Advisory Group to advise the federal government on the Agenda.

Technical Advisory Committee on Tax Measures for Persons with Disabilities:

"Going forward ... Priority should be given to expenditure programs rather than tax measures to target new funding where the need greatest. The [Technical Advisory] Committee recognizes that the development of such programs would involve consultations with provincial and territorial governments and the disability community."

From "Disability Tax Fairness," December 2004

MEDIUM-TERM—3–5 YEARS

1. Explore a further role for the federal government in addressing poverty by meeting individual costs of disability through an expenditure program, perhaps modelled after the National Child Benefit.
2. Integrate the Caregiver Agenda into a Framework for Investment in Disability Supports.

MEASURING SUCCESS

Governments have expressed a commitment to act. We recommend the following four targets for measuring success of this agenda over a 5–10 year period.

1. **Reduce by half the annual income gap between Canadians with and without disabilities**—This would mean increasing the average personal incomes of people with disabilities who have incomes to $26,500 from $22,200 (in 2001 constant dollars). The average income for non-disabled Canadians is $30,800.
2. **Reduce by half the poverty rate of adults with disabilities**—This would mean reducing the prevalence rate of working-age people with disabilities who are living below Statistics Canada's low income cut-off from the current 15% to 11%. The poverty rate for non-disabled Canadians is 6.6%.
3. **Reduce by half the labour-market participation gap between Canadians with and without disabilities**—This would mean increasing the employment rate for people with disabilities to 61% from the current 44%. This would still be well below the employment rate for non-disabled Canadians of 78%, but would signal a major improvement.
4. **Reduce by half the non-reimbursed costs faced by persons with disabilities.**

These are reasonable targets. They are achievable. Canadians with disabilities deserve nothing less.

Federal-Provincial-Territorial Ministers of Social Services

"Ministers ... agreed to jointly develop a strategy for investments in disability programs, with both short and long-term options. Ministers committed to advancing issues that are important to Canadians with disabilities, including the three building blocks of In Unison—disability supports, income, and employment."

From News Release of Federal-Provincial-Territorial Meeting of Ministers Responsible for Social Services, November 2, 2004.

ENDNOTES

1. Ministers commissioned the Canadian Council on Social Development (CCSD) to prepare the study. See CCSD, "Supports and Services for Adults and children Age 5–14 with Disabilities in Canada: An analysis of needs and gaps," Ottawa, December 2004.

2. See Cameron Crawford, "Unmet Needs for Disability Supports." Toronto: The Roeher Institute, January 2005.

3. See Cameron Crawford, "Non-Reimbursed Costs of Disability-Specific Supports: Technical Paper." Toronto: The Roeher Institute, January 2005.

4. All provincial/territorial governments signed the Accord except for Quebec, which agreed to the principles and intent of the agreement.

CHAPTER 18

Economic Gender Equality Indicators 2000

Warren Clark

Gender equality has been identified as a priority for countries around the world. Women are making gains, but persistent disparities exist between women and men. The gender equality indicators presented here were developed in conjunction with Status of Women Canada to measure the balance of the experiences of Canadian women and men in three domains: income, work, and learning. This is the second edition of the indicators. The first was released by the Federal-Provincial/Territorial Ministers Responsible for the Status of Women in October 1997.[1]

The gender equality indexes use ratios of women to men to show the differences between the sexes for a given measure of equality. A ratio of 1.0 means women and men are equal. An index above or below 1.0 indicates inequality or imbalance for that measure: below 1.0, women have less than men; above 1.0, they have more. A gap that is closing over time, converging on 1.0, may result from changes in women's situation, or in men's situation, or both.

DOMAIN: INCOME

Traditionally, gender imbalances in income have been measured by comparing the full-time, full-year earnings of women and men. This is a limited approach because women more often work part-time or part-year than men, making their sources of income more varied and less concentrated on earnings. The income indexes used here recognize all income and earnings of women and men, regardless of their employment status.

DOMAIN: WORK

The decisions people make about dividing their time among work, family, and leisure have numerous implications. Work performed by women is often invisible to current measures of economic progress because only goods and services exchanged for pay are included. Unpaid work—the vast majority of which is still performed by women—is not counted. As everyone has the same amount of time every day, time spent doing paid and unpaid work provides another measure of equality.

Paid work is work performed for remuneration, whether in a separate workplace or at home, and includes wages, salaries, and income from self-employment. Unpaid activities are classified as *unpaid work* when the goods or services produced could have been purchased in the market. For example, unpaid work includes meal preparation, since a meal could be bought at a restaurant; likewise, childcare or elder care are included, because these services could be purchased from day-care centres or retirement homes. In contrast, someone else cannot sleep, learn and travel to and from work for another person, so these activities are not classified as unpaid work.[2]

DOMAIN: LEARNING

Education has been and continues to be a critical element in economic well-being. Not only must people be well-educated when they first enter the labour market, they continually need to learn new skills to take advantage of new opportunities as they arise. These indicators assess the gender balance in university education and work-related training as well as women's return on their investment in education.

INCOME

Total Income Index

The total income index compares the average total income of women and men.[3] In recent years, the total income index has increased, indicating that the gap in total income between genders is narrowing. In 1991, the average total income for Canadian women aged 15 or over was about

$18,000 compared with $30,900 for men. The total income equality index for that year was 0.58, meaning that overall women received about 58% as much income as men (see Figure 18.1).

Figure 18.1: Gender Equality Indexes for Total Income, Total After-tax Income and Total Earnings

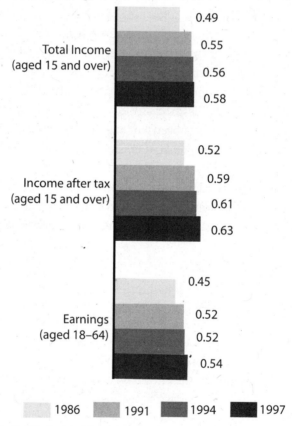

Total Income
(aged 15 and over)
0.49
0.55
0.56
0.58

Income after tax
(aged 15 and over)
0.52
0.59
0.61
0.63

Earnings
(aged 18–64)
0.45
0.52
0.52
0.54

1986 1991 1994 1997

Source: Statistics Canada, Survey of Consumer Finances.

Total After-tax Income Index

The Canadian income tax system is a progressive one, allowing those with less income to keep proportionately more of their money.[4] Because women's income is lower than men's, the total after-tax income index is higher than the total income index. In 1997, the after-tax income index stood at 0.63, up from 0.61 in 1994 (see Figure 18.1).

TOTAL EARNINGS INDEX

This index compares the earnings of women and men aged 18 to 64 and includes those who have no earnings for various reasons (for example, unemployment, disability or full-time child rearing at home). The index includes earnings from part-time work, where women predominate. For this reason, it is lower than the full-time, full-year wage ratio that is often used to measure the wage gap. In 1991, women earned $16,300 compared with $29,900 for men, resulting in a total earnings index of 0.54. Like the other income indexes, the imbalance in earnings between women and men has declined since 1986 (see Figure 18.1).

ANALYZING THE GENDER GAPS

Gender differences in income and earnings may be accounted for in part by women's concentration in part-time work and low-paying occupations; women's overrepresentation among lone parents; and women's overrepresentation among seniors who have low earnings. Calculations were made to account for these and other socio-demographic differences.[5] In 1997, these adjustments reduced the gender gap by seven percentage points in after-tax income and eight percentage points in earnings (see Figure 18.2).[6]

Figure 18.2 Gender Equality Indexes for Income After-tax and Earnings, before and after Accounting for Socio-demographic Factors, 1997

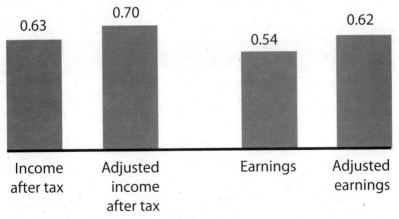

| Income after tax | Adjusted income after tax | Earnings | Adjusted earnings |

0.63   0.70   0.54   0.62

Income after tax   Adjusted income after tax   Earnings   Adjusted earnings

Source: Statistics Canada, Survey of Consumer Finances.

WORK

Total Workload Index

The concept of total workload encompasses both paid work and un-paid work of economic value. In 1998, Canadian women aged 15 and over spent 7.8 hours per day working at paid or unpaid work while men spent 7.5 hours working. The total workload index was 1.04 in 1998, down from 1.08 in 1986. While the gap is shrinking, women work an average of about 15 minutes more per day than men. This imbalance in total work seems to be greatest for young women aged 15 to 24 (1.18) and for senior women (1.11), while women aged 45 to 54 experience near equity (1.01) (see Figure 18.3 and Table 18.1).

Figure 18.3: Gender Equality Index for Total Workload

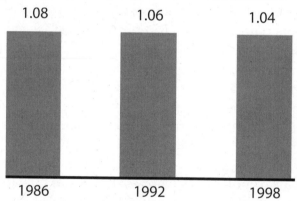

Source: Statistics Canada, General Social Survey

Table 18.1: Gender Equality Index for Workload, by Age Group, 1998

Age of respondent	Total workload index	Paid work index	Unpaid work index
15 and over	1.04	0.62	1.56
15–24	1.18	0.80	1.74
25–34	1.03	0.63	1.75
35–44	1.02	0.60	1.67
45–54	1.01	0.65	1.56
55–64	1.06	0.59	1.42
65+	1.11	0.39	1.19

Source: Statistics Canada, General Social Survey.

Paid Work and Unpaid Work Indexes

Men still spend much more time than women in paid work activities while women spend more time in unpaid work activities. While the gender gap in both paid and unpaid work remains substantial, it declined between 1986 and 1998 (see Figure 18.4).

Figure 18.4: Gender Equality Index for Paid and Unpaid Work

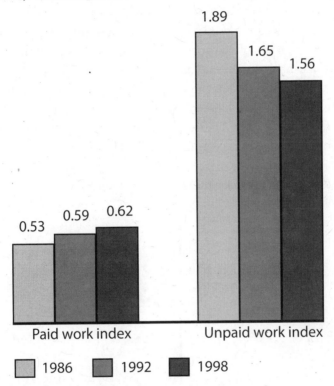

Source: Statistics Canada, General Social Survey

Paid and Unpaid Work Ratios by Household Structure

The distribution of paid and unpaid work between women and men varies with the presence of young children and multiple earners in a household. Separate work indexes were calculated for women and men aged 20 to 44 who are employed full-time. Three household categories of individuals were examined: dual-earners (both spouses employed full-time) with young children (children under age six); primary-earners (two-parent households, other spouse not working full-time) with young children; and earners without young children.

In both 1992 and 1998, women devoted less time to paid and more time to unpaid work, regardless of the household structure. For dual-earners with young children, the differences in paid work between women and men declined. In contrast, the index fell from 0.91 to 0.85 for primary-earners, suggesting that the imbalance is increasing. The change to the imbalance for earners with no young children was very slight. However, because few women are primary-earners with young children, the estimates have high sampling variability. This in turn results in no statistically significant change in the paid work index (see Figure 18.5).

The unpaid work index shows that, over time, the imbalance between women and men has declined for both dual- and primary-earners with young children. The index for earners without young children was about the same in 1998 as in 1992 (see Figure 18.6).

Figure 18.5: Paid Work Index for Women and Men Aged 20–44, Employed Full-time

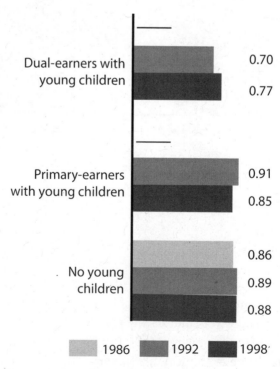

Figure 18.6: Unpaid Work Index for Women Men Aged 20–44, Employed Full-time

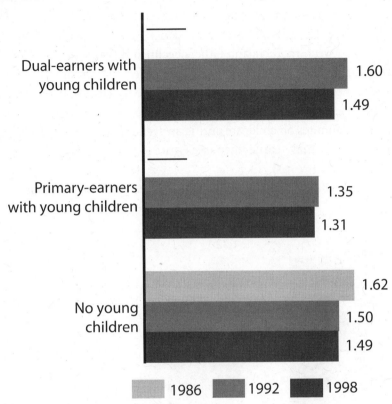

Source: Statistics Canada, General Social Survey.

Beneficiaries of Work

Unpaid work by women and men benefits many people both inside and outside the household. Some unpaid activities such as childcare and volunteer work have obvious beneficiaries while other activities such as housekeeping, or shopping for goods and services or cooking and cleaning, may benefit the entire household or individual members of the household. For the purposes of this comparison, and because work related to children is one of the most important factors affecting women's economic situation when compared with men's, only childcare is examined here.

In 1998, women dual-earners aged 20 to 44 with young children spent more time than men caring for their children on an average day—147 versus 85 minutes. This resulted in an index of 1.72, indicating that women dual-earners spent an estimated 72% more time on childcare than men dual-earners. Though women still spend more time on childcare, the imbalance between mothers and fathers declined between 1992 and 1998. The index for primary-earners in particular declined, from 1.71 to 1.27, which reflects a drop in time spent on childcare activities for women and an increase for men. In 1998, primary-earner women with young children spent 107 minutes on childcare during an average day, compared with 85 minutes for primary-earner men (see Figure 18.7).

Figure 18.7: Childcare Index for Women and Men Aged 20–44, Employed Full-time

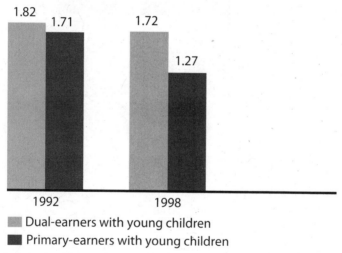

1992

1998

Dual-earners with young children

Primary-earners with young children

Source: Statistics Canada, General Society Survey.

LEARNING

University Degrees Granted Indexes

The university degrees granted index compares the concentration of women in female-dominated, gender-neutral, and male-dominated fields[7] of study for university degrees.

Between 1981 and 1998, more women entered traditionally male-dominated and gender-neutral fields. As a result, the index shows that women's share of degrees granted has increased in all three categories of fields of study, even in female-dominated fields. Although more women are graduating from male-dominated and gender-neutral fields (creating greater gender balance in those fields), more are also graduating from female fields, which accentuates the imbalance in those fields (see Figure 18.8).

Figure 18.8: Gender Equality Indexes for University Degrees Granted

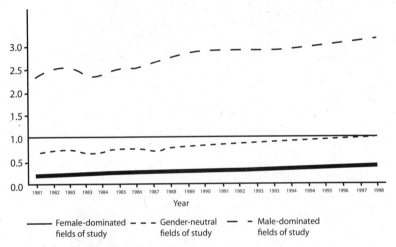

Source: Statistics Canada, University Student Information System (USIS).

Training Indexes

The training participation index shows the extent of employed women's participation in employer-supported training or job-related training.[8] In 1997, employed women were more likely than men to participate in training designed to develop new skills and knowledge (see Figure 18.9). However, the training time index, which compares the actual time spent in training, shows that although women received less employer-supported training than men in 1997, they received more job-related training This suggests that women compensate for less employer-sponsored training by paying for job-related training themselves and by taking it on their own time (see Figure 18.10).

Figure 18.9: Gender Equality Indexes for Training Participation in Canada

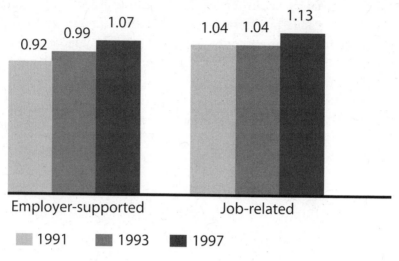

Source: Statistics Canada, General Society Survey.

Figure 18.10: Gender Equality Indexes for Training Hours

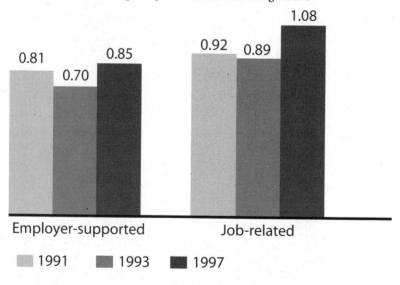

Source: Human Resources Development Canada and Statistics Canada, Adult Education and Training Survey.

Occupational Return on Education Index

This index examines the gender imbalance in the return on invest-ment on university education in terms working in a high-level job.[9] In 1986, 51% of women university graduates worked in high-level jobs compared with 74% of men, and the occupational return index was 0.69. By 1998, 49% of women and 62% of men university graduates aged 25 to 64 were working in high-level jobs, resulting in an index of 0.78. While both men and women university graduates were less likely to be in high-level jobs in 1998, the gap between women's and men's in return on a university education had narrowed (see Figure 18.11).

Figure 18.11: Gender equality index for occupational return on education

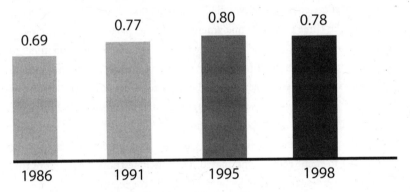

1986   1991   1995   1998

Source: Statistics Canada, Survey of Consumer Finances.

ENDNOTES

1. More information on why these indicators were selected and the conceptual and data issues faced in developing them and how they are intended to stimulate public policy discussion can be found in the original 1997 publica-tion, *Economic Gender Equality Indicators*, available at http://dsp-psd.pwgsc. gc.ca/Collection/SW21-17-1997E.pdf. The historical data in the original pub-lication may differ due to small changes in definitions and revisions to the raw data.

2. The General Social Survey (GSS) estimates of total work include education and related activities and commuting. See *Overview of the Time Use of Cana-dians in 1998.* Statistics Canada Catalogue no. 12Foo8oXIE.

3. Total income includes all income received by an individual during a calendar year from sources such as wages, salaries, self-employment income, investment income, net rental income, pensions, employment insurance, child and spousal support payments and government transfers. Money received from irregular sources, such as windfall gambling gains, inheritances, realized capital gains, or income-in-kind is excluded.

4. Other taxes—such as sales or property taxes—also affect disposable income but are not factored into this index.

5. To eliminate the impact of age, occupation, education, types of employment and family status, average after-tax income and earnings were standardized to show what the pattern would look like if women and men were equally represented in four age groups (15 to 29, 30 to 49, 50 to 64, 65 and over); in 16 occupational categories; in four education groups (less than grade 10, grade 11 to 13, some postsecondary including postsecondary diploma or university degree); in three types of employment (full-time, part-time and no employment); and in two types of family status (a child under 6, no child under 6).

6. For an analysis of gender differences in wages in Canada and the United States in the late 1980s, see Baker, Michael and Nicole Fortin. 2000. *Gender composition and wages: Why is Canada different from the United States?* (Statistics Canada catalogue no. 11F0019MPE, no. 140).

7. Male-dominated fields include those where more than 60% of degrees were granted to men. Female-dominated fields include those where more than 60% of degrees were granted to women. In all other cases, the fields are classified as gender neutral.

8. The training participation index is calculated based on the ratio of the percentage of employed women aged 25 to 49 who took training in the previous 12 months related to the percentage of employed men aged 25 to 49 who did. Separate indexes were calculated for employer-supported training (training paid for or supported by the employer) and job-related training. Job-related training includes both employer-supported training and job-related training paid for by employees themselves.

9. The index is based on the percentage of university degree holders aged 25 to 64 who work in a high-level job. High-level jobs are defined as the three highest categories of the Pineo socio-economic classification of occupations (i.e., self-employed professionals, employed professionals and high-level managers). This classification is based on job income and other characteristics that are related to societal status or prestige. These groups include occupations in health diagnosing, architecture and engineering, social sciences, physical

sciences, elementary, secondary and university teaching and government administration. This scale was originally developed in the 1970s and was updated using 1981 Census data. Further efforts are needed to design a scale using more recent job evaluations.

Part V: Moving Towards Action

Part V provides an agenda for moving on improving the quality of life of Canadians through concerted health promotion action. It outlines some of the barriers to such actions and suggests specific areas for community-based and policy-oriented activity. Particular focus is placed upon the activities of those working in the health sector.

Chapter 20 details some of the barriers to addressing the social determinants of health in Canada. These include the epistemological dominance of positivist approaches to the health sciences, the ideology of individualism prevalent in North America, and the increasing influence of the marketplace on public policy. Various models of public policy provide pathways by which these barriers can be surmounted.

Chapter 21 identifies and suggests means of filling the gaps/needs in Canadian research activity and public policy action on the income and health relationship. It identifies numerous gaps/needs in Canadian research on income and health that fall into five main areas: (i) training and capacity building in addressing income as a health determinant; (ii) developing adequate data and measures; (iii) researching specific substantive health issues areas; (iv) researching specific public policy areas; and (v) developing an understanding of the pathways and mechanisms mediating the income and health relationship.

Chapter 22 outlines an urban health research agenda for health promoters. The authors argue for a participatory urban health research and action agenda with four components: (i) an emphasis on health promotion and the social determinants of health; (ii) community-based participatory research; and (iii) drawing on the lived experience of people to influence (iv) policy analysis and policy change. Urban health researchers and promoters are urged to draw upon new developments in population health and community-based health promotion theory and research to identify and strengthen the roots of urban health through citizen action on public policy.

Chapter 23 outlines what health workers can do to address the social determinants of health. Reasons for Canada's neglect of structural and public policy issues are explored and ways by which public health workers in Canada and elsewhere can help to shift policymakers' and the general public's understanding of the determinants of health are outlined.

Chapter 24 considers how the increasing interest in quality of life can be applied by health promoters in the service of health. Developments in the quality of life field are reviewed and recent findings presented. The focus on the social determinants of health by various agencies and institutions suggests the possibility of a new health promotion movement.

CHAPTER 19

Barriers to Addressing the Social Determinants of Health

Dennis Raphael, Ann Curry-Stevens, Toba Bryant

INTRODUCTION

Despite Canada's reputation as a leader in developing and promoting health promotion and population health concepts, implementation of public policies in support of health has been woefully inadequate [1]. The continuing presence of income, housing, and food insecurity among Canadians has led to Canada being the subject of a series of rebukes from the United Nations for failing to address child and family poverty, discrimination against women and Aboriginal groups, and most recently the crisis of homelessness and housing insecurity [2].

The contrast between words and actions has also been apparent in the area of the social determinants of health [3]. Canada's rich history of policy declarations regarding the importance of public policy for addressing the economic and social conditions underlying health has contributed to the social determinants of health concept [4–6]. Canadians have managed two of the International Commission on the Social Determinants of Health's knowledge hubs—early childhood and globalization and health—and Canadians have made significant contributions to various aspects of the Commission's mandate [7].

Yet on the ground, living conditions continue to deteriorate for many Canadians [2,3,8]. As just one example, Statistics Canada recently reported that over the past 10 years the only group of Canadians showing income gains has been the top 20%, whose incomes have increased substantially [9]. The incomes of the other 80% of Canadian have stagnated. Analyses of Canadian failures to address the social determinants of housing, employment security, food security, social exclusion, and poverty—among others—are available [10].

In this paper we consider two key questions. Considering what is known about these social determinants of health and their importance for promoting the health of Canadians, why does there seem to be so little action undertaken to improve them? And what are the means by which such public policy action in support of health can be brought about?

IDEOLOGY, HEALTH DISCOURSES, AND THE SOCIAL DETERMINANTS OF HEALTH

Most of the public probably believes that academic disciplines such as the health sciences and their applied expressions, public health agencies, and governmental health ministries, carry out their activities based on objective facts drawn from empirical research studies. Within this framework we would understand the health field's current preoccupation with biomedical advances and with what sociologist Nettleton [11] calls the "holy trinity of risk" of tobacco, diet, and physical activity as reflecting the accumulated evidence that these domains are the primary determinants of citizens' health status in developed nations.

Clearly, the pervasive evidence that has accumulated concerning the importance of the social determinants of health does not support this argument [12–15]. There must be more to this neglect of the social determinants of health than meets the eye and indeed, numerous hypotheses are available to inform this analysis. The first concerns the nature—that is, the focus and the analytical tools available—of research and action in the health sciences in general and epidemiology in particular.

The characteristics of traditional health sciences and epidemiological approaches that are problematic have been identified [16–20]. These include (a) reliance on quantitative and statistical approaches to understanding health and its determinants; (b) a tendency towards viewing the sources of health and illness as emanating from individual dispositions and actions rather than resulting from the influence of societal structures; (c) a professed commitment to objectivity or what is termed a non-normative approach to health issues; and (d) a profound depoliticizing of health issues. All of these reflect an adherence to positivist science as the preferred means of understanding health and its determinants [21].

The health sciences in general and epidemiology in particular are a reflection of what has been termed positivist science [21]. Sometimes known as empiricist science, positivist science is based on a natural sciences approach associated with the rise of physics, chemistry, and biology as areas of study. It is focused on the concrete and observable. It has also been called a reductionist approach whereby effort is expended to identify specific variables that can be placed into statistical equations in order to identify putative causes and effects. While positivist science has led to impressive advances in the natural sciences, its application to the fields of the health sciences and other areas of social inquiry has been problematic [18,22].

When applied to the health and social sciences, positivist science generally avoids dealing with aspects of broader environments [23,24]. In the medical field it leads to a focus upon cells, body organs, and bodily systems by biomedical researchers and a focus on behavioural risk factors by health sciences researchers [17,25]. The study of environments and the political, economic, and social forces that shape the quality of these environments is generally neglected [19,26]. The role of politics and political ideology in shaping these environments, therefore, is especially uncommon.

INDIVIDUALISM AND THE SOCIAL DETERMINANTS OF HEALTH

The second barrier to having a social determinants of health approach taken seriously by professionals, the public, and governmental policymakers is the North American commitment to the ideas of individualism and individual responsibility as opposed to communal responsibility [27]. Individualism is the belief that one's place in the social hierarchy—occupational class, income and wealth, and power and prestige as well as the effects of such placement on health and disease status—comes about through one's own efforts [28]. At the very minimum it leads to placing the locus of responsibility for one's health status within the motivations and behaviours of the individual rather than health status being a result of how a society organizes its distribution of a variety of resources.

Individualism in health has numerous effects in relation to the social determinants of health. First, it leads to a strong bias towards understanding health problems as individual problems rather than societal ones. Second, it specifies the cause of the health problem as residing within faulty biomedical markers, specific individual motivations, and risk behaviours that are somehow under individual control. Third, it specifies that improving health will result from modifying these markers, motivations, and behaviours. Fourth, it says little about reorganizing society and its structure in the service of health. Fifth, it says even less about how such societal structures could be modified.

INCREASING MARKET ORIENTATION OF CANADIAN SOCIETY

Finally, the increasing market orientation of Canadian society weakens support for a social determinants of health approach to promoting health [29–31]. The rise of capitalism and the market economy grew in tandem with a strong belief in individualism and the ability of the individual to control one's destiny [32]. The uncritical belief in this ideology was associated with the rise of market-oriented societies that saw little role for governmental or State intervention in the marketplace and in the provision of various forms of security for its citizens.

The rise of differing forms of welfare states in Europe during the 19th century was a response to these excesses of laissez-faire capitalism [32]. In continental Europe a conservative form of the welfare state arose whose main concern was with reducing unrest and promoting a modicum of security for citizens.

In Scandinavia the social democratic welfare state arose, which saw active promotion of equality and human rights and the provision of citizen security across the life span [33]. The third form of the welfare state—the liberal—was the weakest of all and Canada falls within this group. In the liberal welfare state the dominant ideological inspiration is *Liberty* achieved through minimizing governmental interventions, and minimizing so-called "disincentives to work" such as social programs and supports.

Eikermo and Bambra provide an overview of some key welfare state concepts that are especially relevant for the analysis of state receptivity to social determinants of health concepts [34]. These include *decommodification*: "The extent to which individuals and families can maintain a normal and socially acceptable standard of living regardless of their market performance" (p. 4); *defamilisation*: "the degree to which individual adults can uphold a socially acceptable standard of living independently of family relationships, either through paid work or through social security provisions" (p. 4); and *welfare state retrenchment*, which refers to the political backlash that led to welfare state reforms and cuts to social expenditure and usually involved increased privatization and marketization of health and social services.

It is the liberal welfare states—of which Canada, the USA, the UK, Ireland, Australia, and New Zealand are the usual examples—where the degree of decommodification and defamilisation is usually the lowest and the extent of welfare state retrenchment has been the highest.

Therefore, the liberal welfare state and its associated ideology provide barren soil for a well-developed social determinants of health approach.

UNDERSTANDING POLICY CHANGE

Another key issue is the policy change process in Canada and other developed nations. There are varying approaches to understanding the policy change process [35].

Pluralist View

The pluralist view is that public policy decisions result from governments and other policymakers choosing public policy directions based on the competition of ideas in the public arena [35]. This competition of ideas, according to this view, is facilitated by various interest groups who lobby governments to accept their position. Pluralists recognize that there may not be a level playing held in these lobbying attempts, with political, economic, and social elites having an upper hand. Nevertheless the pluralist approach assumes that the governmental policymaking process is generally open and those with the better ideas will come to see their views adopted by governments.

The pluralist view argues therefore that advocates of the social determinants of health view need to get organized and have their voices heard by policymakers. Ongoing consciousness raising, advocacy, and lobbying and building coalitions will achieve policy change (Table 20.1).

Table 19.1: Policy Options to Support the Social Determinants of Health

Policies to reduce the incidence of poverty
Raise the minimum wage to a living wage
Improve pay equity
Restore and improve income supports for those unable to gain employment
Provide a guaranteed minimum income
Policies to reduce social exclusion
Enforce legislation that protects the rights of minority groups, particularly concerning employment rights and anti-discrimination
Ensure that families have sufficient income to provide their children with the means of attaining healthy development
Reduce inequalities in income and wealth within the population, through progressive taxation of income and inherited wealth
Assure access to educational, training, and employment opportunities, especially for those such as the long-term unemployed
Remove barriers to health and social services, which will involve understanding where and why such barriers exist
Provide adequate follow-up support for those leaving institutional care
Create housing policies that provide enough affordable housing of reasonable standard
Institute employment policies that preserve and create jobs
Direct attention to the health needs of immigrants and to the unfavourable socio-economic position of many groups, including the particular difficulties many New Canadians face in accessing health and other care services
Policies to restore and enhance Canada's social infrastructure
Restore health and service program spending to the average level of OECD nations
Develop a national housing strategy and allocate an additional 1% of federal spending for affordable housing
Provide a national day care program
Provide a national pharmacare program
Restore eligibility and level of employment benefits to previous levels
Require that provincial social assistance programs are accessible and funded at levels to assure health
Assure that supports are available to support Canadians through critical life transitions [36, p. 349,351]

Source: Raphael, D. (2004). (ed.) Social determinants of health: Canadian Perspectives, pp. 349-350. Toronto: CSPI

The Materialist View

The materialist view is that governments in capitalist societies such as Canada enact policies that serve the interests of economic elites [35]. These elites are the owners and managers of large corporations whose primary goals are to maximize profits, provide growing profits to shareholders, and institute public policies that keep business costs down. These interests are also likely to lobby for minimal governmental intervention in business practices and to resist business regulation and progressive labour legislation.

The materialist model suggests organizing the population to oppose and defeat the powerful interests that influence governments to maintain inequality [37]. These defeats can occur in the workplace through greater union organizing and the promotion of class solidarity. These defeats can occur in the electoral and parliamentary arena by the ascendance of working-class power.

This can be achieved by restoring programs and services and reintroducing more progressive income tax rates. Independent unions are a necessity, as is legislation that strengthens the ability of workers to organize. Re-regulating many industries would reverse current trends towards the concentration of power and wealth. Internationally, the development and enforcement of agreements to provide adequate working and living standards that would support and promote health and well-being across national barriers is essential.

THE WAY FORWARD

Such an analysis suggests that what is necessary to promote governmental receptivity to the social determinants of health concept is the building of social and political movements in support of health. In the UK such activity may have contributed to the election of a government whose receptivity to these ideas is certainly greater than is the case in Canada and the USA.

Educate

There are hundreds—if not thousands—of Canadians whose occupations are concerned with the health of the public. These workers could take advantage of the citizenry's continuing concern with health and the wealth of evidence of the importance of the social determinants of health to begin offering an alternative message to the dominant biomedical and lifestyle discourse. At a minimum health promoters can carry out—and publicize the findings from—critical analysis of the social determinants of health and disease. This is not a question of being subversive—it is rather a simple matter of information and knowledge transfer.

Motivate

Health researchers and workers can shift public, professional, and policymakers' focus on the dominant biomedical and lifestyle health paradigms to a social determinants of health perspective by collecting and presenting stories about the impact social determinants of health have on people's lives. Ethnographic and qualitative approaches to individual and community health produce vivid illustrations of the importance of these issues for people's health and well-being [38]. There is some indication that policymakers—and certainly the media—may be responsive to such forms of evidence [39,40]. In Canada, such research clearly constitutes a small proportion of public health and health services research [41].

Activate

The final role is the most important but potentially the most difficult: supporting political action in support of health. There is increasing evidence that the quality of any number of social determinants of health within a jurisdiction is shaped by the political ideology of governing parties. It is no accident that nations where the quality of the social determinants of health is high have had greater rule by social democratic parties of the left. Indeed, among developed nations, left-cabinet share in national governments is the best predictor of child poverty rates which itself is associated with extent of government social transfers [42]. Nations with a larger left-cabinet share from 1946 to the 1990s had the lowest child poverty rates and highest social expenditures; nations with less left-share had the highest poverty rates and lowest social expenditures. Canada, like the other liberal nations of New Zealand, Ireland, the UK, and the USA, was among the lowest nations in left federal cabinet share (0%) and among the highest in child poverty rates (15%) in the 1990s (providing a poor poverty standing of 19th of 26 OECD nations).

It has also been documented that poverty rates and government support in favour of health—the extent of government transfers—is higher when the popular vote is more directly translated into political representation through proportional representation [43]. Canada does not have proportional representation—the lack of which is associated with higher poverty rates and less government action in support of health. Proportional representation is important because it provides for an ongoing influence of left-parties regardless of which party forms the government.

The social determinants of health concept can help make the links between government policy, the market, and the health and well-being of citizens in Canada and elsewhere. There are potent barriers, however, to such actions and this is especially the case in nations identified as liberal welfare states. We hope this article can assist in recognizing and surmounting these barriers.

REFERENCES

1. Canadian Population Health Initiative. Canadian population health initiative brief to the commission on the future of health care in Canada. Ottawa: CPHI; 2002.

2. Raphael, D. Poverty and policy in Canada: Implications for health and quality of life. Toronto: Canadian Scholars' Press Inc.; 2007.

3. Raphael, D. Addressing health inequalities in Canada: Little attention, inadequate action, limited success. In: Pederson, A., Rootman, I., O'Neill, M., Dupéré, S., editors. Health promotion in Canada: Critical perspectives. Toronto: Canadian Scholars' Press Inc.; 2007.

4. Epp, J. Achieving health for all: A framework for health promotion. Ottawa, Canada: Health and Welfare Canada; 1986.

5. Lalonde, M. A new perspective on the health of Canadians: A working document. Ottawa: Health and Welfare Canada; 1974.

6. Health Canada. The population health template: Key elements and actions that define a population health approach. Ottawa: Strategic policy directorate, population and public health branch. Health Canada; 2001.

7. World Health Organization. Commission on the social determinants of health. Geneva: World Health Organization; 2008.

8. United Way of Greater Toronto, Canadian Council on Social Development. A decade of decline: Poverty and income inequality in the city of Toronto in the 1990s. Toronto: Canadian Council on Social Development and United Way of Greater Toronto; 2002.

9. Murphy, B. Roberts, P. Wolfson, M. High income Canadians. Perspectives on Labour and Income 2007;(September):5–17.

10. Raphael, D. editor. Social determinants of health: Canadian perspectives. 2nd ed. Toronto: Canadian Scholars' Press Inc.; 2008.

11. Nettleton, S., Surveillance, health promotion and the formation of a risk identity. In: Sidell, M., Jones, L., Katz, J., Peberdy, A., editors. Debates and dilemmas in promoting health. London, UK: Open University Press; 1997, p. 314–24.

12. Davey Smith, G. editor. Inequalities in health: Life course perspectives. Bristol, UK: Policy Press; 2003.

13. Marmot, M., Wilkinson, R. Social determinants of health. 2nd ed. Oxford, UK: Oxford University Press; 2006.

14. Raphael, D. editor. Social determinants of health: Canadian perspectives. Toronto: Canadian Scholars Press Inc.; 2004.

15. Wilkinson, R., Marmot, M. Social determinants of health: The solid facts. Copenhagen, Denmark: World Health Organization, European Office; 2003.

16. Tesh, S. Hidden arguments: Political ideology and disease prevention policy. New Brunswick, NJ: Rutgers University Press; 1990.

17. Bezruchka, S. Epidemiological approaches. In: Raphael, D., Bryant, T., Rioux, M., editors. Staying alive: Critical perspectives on health, illness, and health care. Toronto: Canadian Scholars Press Inc.; 2006.

18. Raphael, D., Bryant, T. The limitations of population health as a model for a new public health. Health Promotion International 2002;17:189–99.

19. Graham, H. Unequal lives: Health and socioeconomic inequalities. New York: Open University Press; 2007.

20. MacDonald, G., Davies, J. Reflection and vision: proving and improving the promotion of health. In: Davies, J. MacDonald, G. editors. Quality, evidence, and effectiveness in health promotion: Striving for certainties. London, UK: Routledge; 1998, p. 5–18.

21. Wilson, J. Positivism. In: Wilson, D. editor. Social theory. Englewood Cliffs, NJ: Prentice Hall; 1983, p. 11–8.

22. Labonte, R. The population health/health promotion debate in Canada: The politics of explanation, economics and action. Critical Public Health 1997; 7(1–2):7–27.

23. Mills ,C.W. The sociological imagination. New York: Oxford University Press; 1959.

24. Lincoln, Y., Guba, E. Naturalist inquiry. Newbury Park, CA: Sage; 1985.

25. Labonte, R. Health promotion and empowerment: Practice frameworks. Toronto: Centre for Health Promotion and ParticipACTION; 1993.

26. Navarro, V. The politics of health inequalities research in the United States. International Journal of Health Services 2004;34(1):87–99.

27. Hofrichter, R. The politics of health inequities: Contested terrain. In: Health and social justice: A reader on ideology, and inequity in the distribution of disease. San Francisco: Jossey Bass; 2003.

28. Travers, K.D. Reducing inequities through participatory research and community empowerment. Health Education and Behaviour 1997;24(3):344–56.

29. Teeple, G. Globalization and the decline of social reform: Into the twenty-first century. Aurora, Ontario: Garamond Press; 2000.

30. Coburn, D. Beyond the income inequality hypothesis: Globalization, neo-liberalism, and health inequalities. Social Science & Medicine 2004;58:41–56.

31. Scarth, T. editor. Hell and high water: An assessment of Paul Martin's record and implications for the future. Ottawa: Canadian Centre for Policy Alternatives; 2004.

32. Esping-Andersen, G. The three worlds of welfare capitalism. Princeton, NJ: Princeton University Press; 1990.

33. Esping-Andersen, G. Politics against markets: The social democratic road to power. Princeton, NJ: Princeton University Press; 1985.

34. Eikemo, T.A., Bambra, C. The welfare state: A glossary for public health. Journal of Epidemiology and Community Health 2008;62(1):3–6.

35. Brooks, S., Miljan, L. Theories of public policy. In: Brooks, S. Miljan, L. editors. Public policy in Canada: An introduction. Toronto: Oxford University Press; 2003.

36. Raphael, D., Curry-Stevens, A. Addressing and surmounting the political and social barriers to health. In: Raphael, D. editor. Social determinants of health: Canadian perspectives. Toronto: Canadian Scholars Press Inc.; 2004.

37. Wright, E.O. The class analysis of poverty. In: Wright, E.O. editor. Interrogating inequality. New York: Verso; 1994, p. 32–50.

38. Popay, I., Williams, G.H., editors. Researching the People's Health, Routledge. London, UK: Routledge; 1994.

39. Bryant, T. Role of knowledge in public health and health promotion policy change. Health Promotion International 2002;17(1):89–98.

40. Whitehead, M., Petticrew, M., Graham, H., Macintyre, S.J., Bambra, C., Egan, M. Evidence for public health policy on inequalities. Part 2. Assembling the evidence jigsaw. Journal of Epidemiology and Community Health 2004;58(10):817–21.

41. Raphael, D., Macdonald, J., Labonte, R., Colman, R., Hayward, K., Torgerson, R. Researching income and income distribution as a determinant of health in Canada: Gaps between theoretical knowledge, research practice, and policy implementation. Health Policy 2004;72:217–32.

42. Rainwater, L., Smeeding, T.M. Poor kids in a rich country: America's children in comparative perspective. New York: Russell Sage Foundation; 2003.

43. Alesina, A., Glaeser, E.L. Fighting poverty in the US and Europe: A world of difference. Toronto: Oxford University Press; 2004.

CHAPTER 20

Income and Health in Canada

Dennis Raphael, Ronald Labonte, Ronald Colman, Karen Hayward, Renee Torgerson, and Jennifer Macdonald

Canada has been a leader in conceptualizing societal determinants of health such as income and its distribution.[1] Concepts developed by the Canadian Institute for Advanced Research, Health Canada, and the Canadian Public Health Association—as three examples—have influenced policy developments around the world.[2] But there is increasing evidence that Canada is failing to apply its own population health concepts in health research.[3] There is also concern that Canada has fallen well behind other nations in applying research findings related to income and its distribution towards policy development.[4-8] The result is a deteriorating public policy environment that increasingly focuses on "lifestyle" and biomedical approaches to understanding and promoting health.[9]

These issues were recognized by the Canadian Institutes of Health Research (CIHR)'s Institute of Population and Public Health (IPPH), a funding agency for health research in Canada. In response to an IPPH call for analyses of how Canadian researchers were responding to emerging health research and health policy needs, we carried out an environmental scan and analysis of how income is considered in health research. The goals of our research were to (a) identify and evaluate gaps/needs in Canadian research into the role that income and its distribution play in Canadians' population health; and (b) recommend means of filling these gaps and meeting these needs.

The specific findings on how Canadian researchers conceptualize income and its distribution as being relevant to health have been published elsewhere.[10] To summarize, these analyses identified the following specific shortcomings: (a) weak conceptualization of how income and its distribution contribute to population health; (b) few longitudinal studies of the effects of income-related issues upon health across the life-span; (c) little interdisciplinary work in the areas of pathways that create and then mediate the income and health relationship; and (d) general neglect of the policy implications of the income and health relationship that could be used to improve population health. The full, detailed final report is available.[11]

Little evidence was seen of work that addresses the political, economic, and social forces that determine how income is distributed within the population. A particularly important area requiring more emphasis is how income and its distribution interact with the presence of social infrastructure, such as public services, to influence health. These are issues that require collaboration with and contribution from social science disciplines such as economics, political science, political economy, sociology, and policy studies. Canadian work fell well below the bar established by leading researchers in the UK and Finland, nations where income and its effects on health are on the public policy agenda.

METHODS

Environmental Scan

In the first part of the study, we identified the total sample of 241 Canadian studies from 1995 to 2002 that applied any one indicator of income, income distribution, socio-economic status, poverty status or other related measure to explain the health outcomes of individuals or populations. We also identified 40 UK and 40 Finnish studies that appeared to us to exemplify the most advanced research in understanding the relationship of income and its distribution to health. Each study was carefully reviewed and coded along a number of conceptual and methodological taxonomies. Further details on the general methods and reliability of ratings are available.[11]

Identification of Gaps and Opportunities

In the second component of the study, the research team identified needs and gaps (combined into a common category) and opportunities on the basis of the literature review, interviews with informants and input from advisory committee members over the course of the research. These gaps/needs were reviewed, modified and then rated by advisory committee members. The members reviewed and discussed the findings of the scan, the research team's comparison of the findings with the exemplary UK and Finnish studies, and the analysis of the interviews with key informants within the context of the priorities of CIHR's IPPH.

More specifically, research team and advisory committee members were in contact across the duration of the study. The committees at each location formally met three times over the course of the study. The first meeting drew upon their collected expertise to identify researchers and research on income and health not easily located in the available academic literature. The second meeting reviewed progress at the halfway point and discussed emerging findings and future directions. The third meeting—and the focus of this article—saw the identification and rating of various measures of filling identified gaps/needs.

FINDINGS

Table 21.1 provides the 31 gaps/needs identified as a result of these activities. The breadth of the list suggests that much can be done to achieve an advanced research agenda of how income and its distribution influence population health in Canada.

Advisory committee members saw little evidence of penetration of emerging population health concepts into most health research in Canada. Instead, emphasis is on traditional risk factor epidemiology with its individualized approach. Social science concepts—concerned with how societal structures shape differential access to health-enhancing opportunities—rarely intrude into most health research, a point noted in the *Canadian Journal of Public Health* and elsewhere.[12-14] Longitudinal data sets allowing analyses of life-course influences upon health are rare. Linked databases are even rarer in Canada. We discuss each cluster of gaps/needs in turn.

Table 20.1: Gaps/Needs Identified through the Environmental Scan and Informant Interviews, and Validated by the Regional Advisory Committees

---

Training/Capacity Building

1. Training in advance conceptualizations, critical perspectives and interdisciplinary work.
2. Applying a common language that conceptualizes values and strengthens the political will to action.
3. Addressing poverty and income inequality as part of health care and public health practice.

Data and Measures

4. Creating longitudinal data and systems for collecting these data.
5. Incorporating measures of socio-economic status, including education and occupational status, into all health research data collection.
   - Including these measures as part of routine data collection related to births, deaths and hospitalizations.
   - Developing and collecting measures of accumulated wealth.
6. Establishing data linkages
   - Routinely linking health data to health-related data sets, such as census and surveys.
   - Data-sharing across provinces.
   - Blending Statistics Canada's Survey of Consumer Finance with available health information.
7. Resolving problems associated with privacy and confidentiality to ensure that there is access to information.
8. Applying research measures such as self-reported health and other measures used in the SF36 (an international health survey).
9. Collecting more surveillance data on health in relation to income and social status.
10. Applying more regional and subregional analysis, for example taking advantage of the new health region analysis available in the Canadian Community Health Survey to expose health differentials.

Specific Health Research Areas

11. Developing a broader understanding of the structural determinants of health.
12. Doing research of the lived experiences of people with low incomes and of how income affects other social determinants of health.
    - More qualitative research uncovering shared social values and subjective information.
13. Creating participatory action research projects that address poverty-related issues.
14. Doing research intervention studies.
    - i.e., What would happen if we increased people's incomes?
    - i.e., What is the impact of intervention x on population y?
15. Performing more research on neighbourhood structure and how it interacts with income and the availability of resources for social infrastructure to influence health, e.g., social capital, and strengthening communities.

16. Carrying out interdisciplinary research involving economists and population health researchers, among many other disciplines.

17. Collecting more information on ethno-racial communities with community participation; linguistically and culturally appropriate measures, survey tools and indices; and integration of alternative cultural paradigms (beyond Eurocentric approaches)

18. Carrying out cost-benefit analysis to explain how poverty affects health status and how it is costly to the health care system.

19. Doing attitudinal research: How does the general public (people who are not poor) view poverty and health? This, in turn, affects the way the public and professionals interact with people who live in poverty and the way services are delivered.

Specific Public Policy Areas

20. Investigating the disconnect between research and health policy (e.g., informing recent initiatives in chronic disease, federal strategies to support "healthy living", heart health work, diabetes strategy, etc.)

21. Carrying out attitudinal research on policy-makers: How do they react to such research, and when/how has the research had some impact?

22. Investigating the thresholds for poverty.
   • How can we develop policy interventions without understanding the impact of the different dimensions of poverty more broadly?
   • What do people need in order to feel as though they can meaningfully participate in society?

23. Doing critical policy analysis that systematically addresses the context, process and content of policies.
   • Understanding the health impact of the public policy process.
   • Understanding political, social and economic forces that influence policy development.

24. Gaining better understanding of the role of media discourses on poverty, inequality and health in the public understanding of and support for ameliorative policies.

25. Learning what macroeconomic and policy interventions maximize reductions in poverty and income inequality.
   • How do certain policies influence poverty incidence and the effect of poverty on health?
   • How do changes in tax policy entitlement to public programs and social goods actually change people's real income rather than command over resources?

26. Gaining better understanding of the role of non-income transfers (tax-funded welfare benefits such as universal health care, education, recreation, etc.) in poverty/health and the income inequality/health relationship.
   • In terms of different income security programs in different countries, what effect do they have on health outcomes across countries/jurisdictions?
   • Look at the associations between measures of income and measures of health at the individual level and how that association differs among countries.

**Pathways/Mechanisms that Mediate the Income
and Health Relationship**

27. Sorting out the process through which income and socio-economic status (SES) variables are associated with health, i.e., How do behavioral and SES risk factors work together to affect health?

28. Understanding the character of societies that are able to buffer the relationship between low income and poor health.

29. Understanding how the poverty cycle creates habitual behaviours and how much of it is responsive to monetary changes.

30. Gathering more information on the effects of people's movement in and out of poverty and the effects of poverty on health over time.

31. Doing better theorization of pathways, developing different research methodologies to do so.

• What are the mechanisms that influence how income influences health?
• What is the relative contribution of life course factors vs. current factors to producing the gradient?

Training and Capacity Building in Addressing Income as a Health Determinant

Advisory committee members were not particularly surprised to see how little penetration there had been of population health concepts into health research. Nor were they surprised to see how little emphasis there was on structural aspects of the income and health relationship among these same researchers.

Developing Adequate Data and Measures

One of the explanations for the current state of Canadian health research into income and health is the lack of well-developed data collection systems that allow complex questions about the determinants of health and illness across the life-span to be answered. There is little consistent effort made to collect socio-demographic data by health authorities, and linkages between health status data and socio-demographic data are virtually non-existent.

Researching Specific Substantive Health Issues

There is limited research being done on understanding the role that broader determinants of health play in population health, and the research that is being done is virtually all quantitative. There is an important need to carry out participatory research studies that can illuminate the lived experiences of Canadians in general and those at risk of poor health in particular. There is also a need for studies that would examine the effects of policy interventions intended to improve the quality of various social determinants of health, such as income. Such studies would require interdisciplinary research involving a range of social scientists.

Researching Specific Public Policy Areas

There is very little research that considers the role that public policy plays in determining health outcomes of Canadians. We need to understand why many current health initiatives are limited to risk factor approaches despite accumulating knowledge of the relatively minor role that lifestyle choices play in health status among populations. There is little critical policy analysis that considers how public policies are created and what impacts they have on the population in general and the vulnerable in particular.

Developing an Understanding of Pathways and Mechanisms Mediating the Income and Health Relationship

As documented in our analyses, explication of the pathways that mediate the income and health relationship is generally undeveloped among health researchers. There are pockets of excellence, but the most striking conclusion is that such analyses are few and far between. These findings are especially surprising considering Canada's perceived leadership in health promotion and population health. Much needs to be done to improve our ability to understand the sources of health in general, and the role that income and its distribution play in health in particular.

CONCLUSIONS AND RECOMMENDATIONS

Our research identified numerous areas in which Canadian research on the role that income and its distribution plays in population health could be enhanced. The particular areas of weakness include the conceptualization of how income and its distribution contribute to population health, lack of longitudinal studies of the impact of income-related issues upon health across the life-span, and lack of linked databases that would allow complex analyses of how income and related issues contribute to health and well-being. There is also little interdisciplinary work that examines the political and economic forces influencing how income is distributed among Canadians.

A lack of interdisciplinary work on the pathways that mediate the income and health relationship also exists, specifically the biological pathways by which issues such as income and its distribution get "under the skin" to influence health. Little work has considered the policy implications of the income and health relationship to improve population health and how these are related to political and economic processes. Indeed, present Canadian policy directions that emphasize individual lifestyle choices and behavioural changes are profoundly at odds with the findings that income and other social determinants of health influence population health.

The media need to be sensitive to these findings. A review of newspaper stories done as part of the needs, gaps and opportunities assessment (NGOA) found that stories involving income and poverty issues in health are usually not based on studies from scientific journals.[11] Rather, they involve coverage of activities by social development or poverty groups that raise the issue in their press releases or press conferences. This is in stark contrast to newspaper stories that report on a daily basis the latest journal findings of how behavioural factors such as diet, physical activity, and tobacco use influence health and disease. IPPH should consider an initiative similar to the WHO-EURO's campaign, Social Determinants of Health: The Solid Facts.[15] IPPH should urge *Horizons, Policy Options,* and other policy-related journals to offer special issues that would report the findings of these NGOAs. This would facilitate dissemination of their results and raise the profile of contextual factors in population health.

The academic, funding and political climate of Canada presents many challenges to researchers pursuing health inequalities research.[16,17] There is a definite need in Canada for a stronger political will to tackle issues relevant to health inequalities.[18] Political will can be influenced by health researchers who consider the social, political, and economic contexts influencing the health of individuals. The primary determinants of political will, however, may be the influence of actions and advocacy by community agencies and various social movements that can draw upon existing bodies of health research focused on these issues.[19-21]

REFERENCES

1. Restrepo, H.E. Introduction. In: *Health Promotion: An Anthology.* Washington DC: Pan American Health Organization, 1996: ix–xi.

2. Raphael, D., Bryant, T. The limitations of population health as a model for a new public health. *Health Promotion Int* 2002;17:189–99.

3. Raphael, D. Health inequalities in Canada: Current discourses and implications for public health action. *Critical Public Health* 2000;10(2):193–216.

4. National Council of Welfare. *Presentation to the Standing Committee on Finance for the 2003 Pre-Budget Consultations.* Ottawa: National Council of Welfare, 2003.

5. National Council of Welfare. *Income for Living?* Ottawa: National Council of Welfare, 2004.

6. National Council of Welfare. *Poverty Profile 2001.* Ottawa: National Council of Welfare, 2004.

7. National Council of Welfare. *From Poverty To Prosperity, Presentation to the Standing Committee on Finance for the 2005 Pre-Budget Consultations.* Ottawa: National Council of Welfare, 2005.

8. Canadian Population Health Initiative. *Canadian Population Health Initiative Brief to the Commission on the Future of Health Care in Canada.* Available at: <http://secure.cihi.ca/cihiweb/en/downloads/cphi_policy_romanowbrief_e.pdf>. Accessed February 20, 2004.

9. Raphael, D. Barriers to addressing the determinants of health: Public health units and poverty in Ontario, Canada. *Health Promotion Int* 2003;18:397–405.

10. Raphael, D., Macdonald, J., Labonte, R., Colman, R., Hayward, K., Torgerson, R. Researching income and income distribution as a determinant of health in Canada: Gaps between theoretical knowledge, research practice, and policy implementation. *Health Policy* 2004; 72:217–32.

11. Raphael, D., Colman, R., Labonte, R., MacDonald, J., Torgeson, R., Hayward, K. *Income, Health and Disease in Canada: Current State of Knowledge, Information Gaps and Areas of Needed Inquiry.* York University. 2001–2002. Available at: <http://www.atkinson.yorku.ca/draphael.>.

12. Frohlich, K.L., Mykhalovskiy, E., Miller, F., Daniel, M. Advancing the population health agenda: Encouraging the integration of social theory into population health research and practice. *Can J Public Health* 2004;95(5):392–5.

13. Shaw, M. Editorial: The accidental epidemiologist. *Int J Epidemiol* 2002;31: 523–26.

14. Labonte, R., Polanyi, M., Muhajarine, N., McIntosh, T., Williams, A. Beyond the divides: towards critical population health research. *Critical Public Health* 2005;15(1):5–17.

15. Wilkinson, R., Marmot, M. *Social Determinants of Health: The Solid Facts.* World Health Organization, European Office, 2003. Available at: <http://www.euro.who.int/document/e81384.pdf>.

16. Bryant, T. Politics, public policy and population health. In: Raphael, D., Bryant, T., Rioux, M., (Eds.), *Staying Alive: Critical Perspectives on Health, Illness, and Health Care.* Toronto: Canadian Scholars Press, 2006:193–216.

17. Raphael, D., Bryant, T. Public health concerns in Canada, USA, UK, and Sweden: exploring the gaps between knowledge and action in promoting population health. In: Raphael, D. Bryant, T. Rioux, M. (Eds.), *Staying Alive: Critical Perspectives on Health, Illness, and Health Care.* Toronto: Canadian Scholars Press, 2006.

18. Coburn, D. Health and health care: a political economy perspective. In: Raphael D., Bryant, T., Rioux, M., (Eds.), *Staying Alive: Critical Perspectives on Health, Illness, and Health Care.* Toronto: Canadian Scholars Press, 2006:59–84.

19. Hofrichter, R. The politics of health inequities: Contested terrain. *Health and Social Justice: A Reader on Ideology, and Inequity in the Distribution of Disease.* San Francisco: Jossey Bass, 2003.

20. Raphael, D., Bryant, T., Rioux, M., (Eds.). *Staying Alive: Critical Perspectives on Health, Illness, and Health Care.* Toronto: Canadian Scholars Press, 2006.

21. Raphael, D., Curry-Stevens, A. Addressing and surmounting the political and social barriers to health. In: Raphael, D. (Ed.). *Social Determinants of Health: Canadian Perspectives.* Toronto: Canadian Scholars Press, 2004.

CHAPTER 21

Identifying and Strengthening the Structural Roots of Urban Health in Canada

Toba Bryant, Dennis Raphael, and Robb Travers

INTRODUCTION

Health promotion has a long tradition of emphasizing community action to influence the determinants of health. One of health promotion's achievements was the *Healthy Cities Movement*, which emphasized community participation and intersectoral action in support of healthy public policy (Ashton, 1992). The *Belfast Declaration on Healthy Cities* reflects a commitment by European municipal leaders to apply these principles to reduce health inequalities and poverty, promote citizen influence, and address social exclusion (World Health Organization, 2003).

URBAN ISSUES AND URBAN HEALTH IN CANADA

Urban issues are a major concern of Canadian municipal, provincial, and federal policy makers (Government of Canada, 2004). Increasing income inequality and poverty, homelessness and housing insecurity, and social exclusion of racial minorities, new immigrants, and the economically disadvantaged are profoundly important to health (Auger, Raynault, Lessard, & Choinière, 2004; Galabuzi, 2005). The association between these urban issues and urban health comes about through the concept of the social determinants of health (Marmot & Wilkinson, 2006; Raphael, 2004b).

Social determinants of health are the political, economic, and social forces that influence health at the individual, group, community, and population levels (Raphael, 2004a). These factors have as much, if not more, impact on health as do traditional medical and behavioural risk factors (Davey Smith, 2003).

A focus on urban health with a renewed emphasis on the social determinants of health therefore appears timely. Many political, economic, and social challenges—all of which influence people's health—are based in urban communities (Government of Canada, 2004). We outline an urban health research and action agenda of four components: a) an emphasis on health promotion and the social determinants of health; b) carried out through community-based participatory research; c) that explores the lived experience of people; d) to effect policy analysis and change (Figure 22.1).

Figure 21.1: Components of the Urban Health and Action Agenda

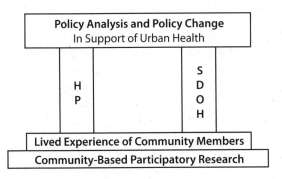

COMPONENT 1: HEALTH PROMOTION AND THE SOCIAL DETERMINANTS OF HEALTH

> *Health promotion is the process of enabling people to increase control over, and to improve, their health* (World Health Organization, 1986).

Health promotion is based on a commitment to improve health and well-being by developing healthy public policy (World Health Organization, 1986). Health promotion has its origins in structural analyses of health issues based on the application of social science methods to health problems (MacDonald & Davies, 1998). The most succinct statement of the principles and values of health promotion is in the Ottawa Charter for Health Promotion (World Health Organization, 1986).

In line with its predominantly structural approach to promoting health, the Charter identifies the prerequisites for health of peace, shelter, education, food, income, a stable ecosystem, sustainable resources, social justice, and equity. Five action areas are outlined: building healthy public policy; creating supportive environments; strengthening community action; developing personal skills; and reorienting health services. Two of these areas are especially relevant to our model: strengthening community action and building healthy public policy. The prerequisites of health are now spoken of as social determinants of health.

COMPONENT 2: COMMUNITY-BASED PARTICIPATORY RESEARCH (CBPR)

> *CBPR holds immense potential for addressing challenging health and social problems, while helping bring about conditions in which communities can recognize and build on their strengths and become full partners in gaining and creating knowledge and mobilizing for change* (Minkler, Wallerstein, & Hall, 2002, p. 20).

CBPR is research that engages community members as research partners to collaboratively tackle community-relevant issues. Studies take place in the community rather than in research labs and offer capacity-building opportunities so skills remain in the community once a study is complete (Parker, Margolis, Eng, & Henriquez-Roldan, 2003). CBPR moves from a model of academic ownership to one of joint ownership with communities (Manson, Garoutte, & Turner Goins, 2004). CBPR also requires an intellectual commitment to look at the day-to-day lived experiences and understandings held by community members (O'Brien Teengs & Travers, 2006).

The five key contributions that CBPR offers to understand and promote community-based health are to:

- provide voice (e.g. power, capacity, control) to communities and their members;
- increase theoretical and practical knowledge about community health;
- improve health through community action;
- identify community issues requiring action; and
- effect political and social change.

Further details concerning each of these contributions of CBPR are available elsewhere (Park, 1993).

COMPONENT 3: LIVED EXPERIENCE OF PEOPLE

> *If public health research is to develop more robust and holistic explanations for patterns of health and illness in contemporary society, and contribute to more appropriate and effective preventive policies, then the key is to utilize and build on lay knowledge—the knowledge that lay people have about illness, health, risk, disability and death* (Williams & Popay, 1997, p. 267).

There are especially compelling theoretical and practical reasons for favoring a lived experience approach. A criticism of traditional approaches to understanding community health is their inability to focus upon the lived experience of people (Bryman, 1988). Lincoln has argued that the most effective way of understanding health-related issues is by discerning individuals' perceptions and constructions of events (Lincoln, 1994). Exploration of the meaning of health and staying healthy among community members provides rich insights that cannot be assessed by traditional approaches (Blaxter, 1990; Popay & Williams, 1994).

This missing piece in health research has been termed interactive knowledge (Park, 1993). Its focus is the meanings and interpretations individuals place on events. Its theoretical bases are phenomenology, symbolic interactionism, and grounded theory (Lincoln & Guba, 1985).

A related form of understanding is critical or reflective knowledge. Critical knowledge is derived from reflection and action on what is right and just. It considers how societal structures and power relations promote inequalities and disenable people.

COMPONENT 4: POLICY ANALYSIS AND CHANGE EMPHASIS

> *Policies shape how money, power and material resources flow through society and therefore affect the determinants of health.*

> *Advocating healthy public policies is the most important strategy we can use to act on the determinants of health* (Canadian Public Health Association, 1996, p. 1).

Thinking about health and its determinants increasingly focuses on the distribution of resources within societies and how these influence health (Raphael, 2003). Also important are government decisions that determine how resources are distributed (Raphael & Curry-Stevens, 2004). For example, social spending—which results in either strong or weak programs in support of health—is shaped by the political ideology of the government of the day, public perceptions towards those in need, and the dominance of particular approaches to evidence deemed legitimate to inform these issues (Bryant, 2006). Government policies—while shaped by prevailing ideologies—can be influenced by citizen action (Esping-Andersen, 1985; Langille, 2004).

CONCLUSION

Our four components provide the analytic tools for working towards these goals of promoting urban health in Canada. They specify the pathways for citizen participation—community-based research and lived experience—in the development and design of healthy cities through healthy public policy development and change. These components give citizens a voice in project and program development and political decisions. These pathways provide opportunities for capacity-building among citizens to develop academic and community research partnerships to address community issues.

REFERENCES

Ashton, J. (1992). *Healthy cities.* New York: Routledge.

Auger, N., Raynault, M., Lessard, R., & Choinière, R. (2004). "Income and health in Canada." In Raphael, D. (Ed.), *Social determinants of health: Canadian perspectives.* Toronto: Canadian Scholars' Press.

Blaxter, M. (1990). *Health and lifestyles.* London UK: Tavistock and Routledge.

Bryant, T. (2006). "Politics, public policy and population health." In Raphael, D., Bryant, T., & Rioux, M. (Eds.), *Staying alive: Critical perspectives on health, illness, and health care.* Toronto: Canadian Scholars Press.

Bryman, A. (1988). *Quantity and quality in social research.* Boston: Unwin Hyman.

Canadian Public Health Association. (1996). *Action statement for health promotion in Canada.* Ottawa: CPHA.

Davey Smith, G. (Ed.). (2003). *Inequalities in health: Life course perspectives.* Bristol UK: Policy Press.

Esping-Andersen, G. (1985). *Politics against markets: The social democratic road to power.* Princeton: Princeton University Press.

Galabuzi, G. E. (2005). *Canada's economic apartheid: The social exclusion of racialized groups in the new century.* Toronto: Canadian Scholars' Press.

Government of Canada. (2004). *Speech from the throne.* Ottawa: Government of Canada.

Langille, D. (2004). "The political determinants of health." In Raphael, D. (Ed.), *Social determinants of health: Canadian perspectives.* Toronto: Canadian Scholars' Press.

Lincoln, Y. (1994). "Sympathetic connections between qualitative research methods and health research." *Qualitative Health Research*, vol. 2, pp. 375–391.

Lincoln, Y., & Guba, E. (1985). *Naturalist inquiry.* Newbury Park CA: Sage.

MacDonald, G., & Davies, J. (1998). "Reflection and vision: Proving and improving the promotion of health." In Davies, J. & MacDonald, G. (Eds.), *Quality, evidence, and effectiveness in health promotion: Striving for certainties.* London, UK: Routledge.

Manson, S. M., Garoutte, E., & Turner Goins, R. (2004). "Access, relevance, and control in the research process: lessons from Indian country." *Journal of Aging and Health*, vol. 16, pp. 58S–77S.

Marmot, M., & Wilkinson, R. (2006). *Social determinants of health* (2nd ed.). Oxford, UK: Oxford University Press.

Minkler, M., Wallerstein, N., & Hall, B. (2002). *Community-based participatory research for health.* San Francisco: Jossey Bass.

O'Brien Teengs, D. & Travers, R. (2006). 'River of life, rapids of change': Understanding HIV vulnerability among two-spirit youth who migrate to Toronto. *Canadian Journal of Aboriginal Community-Based Research*, vol. 1, pp. 17–28.

Park, P. (1993). "What is participatory research? A theoretical and methodological perspective." In Park, P. Brydon-Miller, M., Hall, B., & Jackson, T. (Eds.), *Voices of change: Participatory research in the United States and Canada.* Toronto: Ontario Institute for Studies in Education Press.

Parker, E., Margolis, L. H., Eng, E., & Henriquez-Roldan, C. (2003). "Assessing the capacity of health departments to engage in community-based participatory public health." *American Journal of Public Health*, vol. 93, pp. 472–476.

Popay, J., & Williams, G. H. (Eds.). (1994). *Researching the people's health*. London, UK: Routledge.

Raphael, D. (2003). "A society in decline: The social, economic, and political determinants of health inequalities in the USA." In Hofrichter, R. (Ed.), *Health and social justice: A reader on politics, ideology, and inequity in the distribution of disease*. San Francisco: Jossey Bass.

Raphael, D. (2004a). Introduction to the social determinants of health. In Raphael, D. (Ed.), *Social determinants of health: Canadian perspectives*. Toronto: Canadian Scholars' Press.

Raphael, D. (Ed.). (2004b). *Social determinants of health: Canadian perspectives*. Toronto: Canadian Scholars' Press.

Raphael, D., & Curry-Stevens, A. (2004). "Addressing and surmounting the political and social barriers to health." In D. Raphael (Ed.), *Social determinants of health: Canadian perspectives*. Toronto: Canadian Scholars' Press.

Williams, G., & Popay, J. (1997). Social science and the future of population health. In L. Jones & M. Sidell (Eds.), *The challenge of promoting health*. London, UK: The Open University.

World Health Organization. (1986). *Ottawa charter for health promotion*. Copenhagen WHO European Office. Available: http://www.who.int/hpr/NPH/docs/ottawa_charter_hp.pdf

World Health Organization. (2003). Belfast declaration. Copenhagen: WHO European Office. Available: http://www.healthycitiesbelfast2003.com/Belfast/BelfastDeclarationFinalUK.pdf

CHAPTER 22

Getting Serious about the Social Determinants of Health

Dennis Raphael

INTRODUCTION

Renewed interest in the social determinants of health in Canada and other nations—best illustrated by the WHO's Commission on the Social Determinants of Health (CSDH) (1)—represents yet another cycle of recognition of the importance of structural determinants of health that began in earnest in the 1850s with the writings of Friedrich Engels (2) and Rudolph Virchow (3). For Canadian—and other—public health workers, the calls for renewed focus on early life, education, employment and working conditions, food security, health care services, housing, income and its distribution, the social safety net, social exclusion, and unemployment and employment security (4) produce a déjà vu experience recalling the *Ottawa Charter*'s prerequisites of health: peace, shelter, education, food, income, stable ecosystem, sustainable resources, social justice, and equity (5).

Just as was the case in 1986 with the release of the *Ottawa Charter* and the *Achieving Health for All* report, the CSDH has generated Canadian governmental and institutional activity (6,7). But now, with the benefit of hindsight, it is clear that action upon strengthening the social determinants of health following these 1986 statements was restrained by Canada's joining the UK, the USA, New Zealand, and Australia in a neo-liberal resurgence in public policy approaches that served to effectively squash attempts to restructure society in favour of health (8).

LOOKING BACK AND LOOKING FORWARD

Now some 20+ years later in the midst of neo-liberal-inspired economic globalization, free trade agreements, and continuing government withdrawal from social provision, public health workers in Canada and elsewhere are again being urged to identify and modify the structural determinants of health whose decay during this interim is evident (9). How likely are public health workers to succeed in these efforts? What can we take from the experiences since 1986 to produce activities more likely of success?

THE POLITICAL ECONOMY OF THE SOCIAL DETERMINANTS OF HEALTH

It is becoming increasingly apparent that the quality of numerous social determinants of health such as early childhood, employment security and working conditions, and the social safety net is predicted by whether a nation is identified as a liberal, conservative, or social democratic political economy as described by Gosta Esping-Andersen (10,11).

Nations with what is termed a liberal political economy such as Canada, Ireland, the UK, and the USA have historically seen relatively less government action in support of the social determinants of health; nations with social democratic political economies such as Denmark, Finland, Norway, and Sweden much more so. Nations with conservative political economies such as France, Germany, and the Netherlands fall in the middale (12).

Figure 22.1: Ideological Variations in Forms of the Welfare State

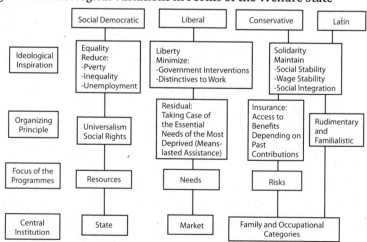

Source: Saint-Arnaud and Bernard (3% Figure 2, p. 503)

Canadian sociologists Saint-Arnaud and Bernard provide a narrative and graphic that succinctly sums up how these differences in political economy come to be related to the quality of the social determinants of health (13). Figure 23.1 lays out the fundamental characteristics of the varying forms of the welfare state in wealthy industrialized nations.

Of particular interest are their guiding principles and dominant institutions. Canada is a liberal welfare state (14). Liberal welfare states provide the least support and security to their citizens. Canadians consider their welfare state to be much superior to that of the USA, but when viewed within an international perspective, Canada's approach is closer to that of the USA than to European welfare states where poverty levels are lower and greater value is placed upon the economic and social security of citizens.

Within liberal welfare states the dominant ideological inspiration is that of liberty, which leads to minimal government intervention in the workings of the marketplace (13). Indeed, such interventions are seen as providing a disincentive to work, thereby breeding "welfare dependence." The results of this ideological inspiration are the meagre benefits provided to those on social assistance in Canada, weak legislative support for the labour movement, undeveloped policies for assisting those with disabilities, and a general reluctance to provide universal services and programmes. Programmes that exist are residual, meaning they exist to provide the most basic needs of the most deprived. Canada, the USA, the UK, and Ireland are the best current exemplars of this form of the welfare state.

Critical social scientists have argued that these liberal welfare states and their ideological characteristics represent the interests of those allied with the central institution of these nations: the market (12,15). It is not an accident that these liberal welfare states have the greatest degree of wealth and income inequality, the weakest safety nets, and the poorest population health (16). These states are prone to cater to the well-off in society who either have interests in the business sector or have come to believe that their interests are best represented by this sector. And it is the business sector in Canada that has most vociferously opposed policies that would reduce poverty, strengthen the social safety net, and improve the lives of the most insecure in Canadian society (17).

The opposite situation is seen among social democratic welfare states. As difficult as it may be for Canadians—and others—to imagine, the ideological inspiration for the central institution of these nations—the State—is the reduction of poverty, inequality, and unemployment. Rather than being concerned with governments meeting the basic needs of the most deprived, the organizing principle here is universalism and providing for the social rights of all citizens.

Denmark, Finland, Norway, and Sweden are the best exemplars of this form of the welfare state. Governments with social democratic political economies are proactive in identifying social problems and issues, and strive to promote economic and social security for their citizens. The outcome of this form of the welfare state has been the virtual elimination of poverty, the striving for gender and social class equity, and the regulation of the market in the service of citizens.

Type of political economy determines societal receptiveness to the concept and policy implications raised by a social determinants of health approach (18). Consider the difficulties Canadian public health workers—and those in other liberal political economies—experience having these broader living-conditions-related issues addressed in Canadian legislatures governed by neo-liberal-oriented political parties (19–21). This is not a problem of evidence, it is a problem of political will (22).

PUBLIC HEALTH ROLES: EDUCATING THE PUBLIC, HEALTH PROFESSIONALS, AND POLICYMAKERS

There are roles that public health workers can play—in addition to their day-to-day efforts to promote health—in promoting healthy public policy in areas related to the social determinants of health. These activities will be especially important—and probably the most contentious—in nations operating under liberal political economies.

Presenting the Solid Facts

In Canada and other nations governed by liberal political economies, the public remains woefully uninformed about the social determinants of health (23–25). The population has also been subject to continuous messaging as to the benefits of a business-oriented laissez-faire approach to governance (8). What this messaging has not included are the societal effects of this approach: increasing income and wealth inequality; persistent poverty; and a relatively poor population health profile (12).

There is no shortage of areas in which public health workers could engage: social determinants of health such as poverty, housing and food insecurity, and social exclusion appear to be the primary antecedents of just about every affliction known to humankind (26,27). My short list of such afflictions includes coronary heart disease, type II diabetes, arthritis, stroke, many forms of cancer, respiratory disease, HIV/AIDS, Alzheimer's, asthma, injuries, death from injuries, mental illness, suicide, emergency room visits, school drop-out, delinquency and crime, unemployment, alienation, distress, and depression.

Telling Stories

Public health workers can shift public, professional, and policymakers' focus on the dominant biomedical and lifestyle health paradigms to a social determinants of health perspective by collecting and presenting stories about the impact social determinants of health have on people's lives. Ethnographic and qualitative approaches to individual and community health produce vivid illustrations of the importance of these issues for people's health and well-being (28). There is some indication that policymakers—and certainly the media—may be responsive to such forms of evidence (29).

Providing Support for Policy Action

The final role is the most important but potentially the most difficult: supporting policy action in support of health. And implicit in such a course of action is recognizing the important role politics play in these activities (30). There is increasing evidence that the quality of any number of social determinants of health within a jurisdiction is shaped by the political ideology of governing parties.

It is no accident that nations where the quality of the social determinants of health is high have had greater rule by social democratic parties of the left. Canada, like the other liberal nations of Ireland, the UK, and the USA is among the lowest nations in rule by left political parties.

It has also been documented that poverty rates and government support in favour of health—the extent of government transfers—is higher when the popular vote is more directly translated into political representation through proportional representation (31). Proportional representation is important because it provides for an ongoing influence of left parties regardless of which party forms the government.

CONCLUSION

A political economy approach recognizes that social democratic-oriented public policies create the conditions necessary for health. These conditions include equitable distribution of wealth and progressive tax policies that create a large middle class, strong programmes that support children, families, and women, and economies that support full employment: "[F]or those wishing to optimize the health of populations by reducing social and income inequalities, it seems advisable to support political forces such as the labour movement and social democratic parties which have traditionally supported larger, more distributive policies" (32, p. 490).

The best means of promoting health through a social determinants of health perspective would involve agencies, organizations, and even government employees navigating the difficult task of informing citizens about the political and economic forces that shape the health of a society.

Once public health has done its task of educating these constituencies, each and any of these groups could then choose to consider political and other means of addressing these issues.

REFERENCES

1. World Health Organization. Commission on the Social Determinants of Health. Geneva, Switzerland: World Health Organization; 2008.

2. Engels, F. The condition of the working class in England. New York: Penguin Classics: 1845/1987.

3. Virchow, R. Collected essays on public health and epidemiology. Cambridge, UK: Science History Publications; 1848/1985.

4. Raphael, D. editor. Social determinants of health: Canadian perspectives. Toronto: Canadian Scholars' Press; 2004.

5. World Health Organization. Ottawa Charter for Health Promotion. Geneva, Switzerland: World Health Organization European Office; 1986.

6. Public Health Agency of Canada and Health Systems Knowledge Network. Crossing sectors: experiences in intersectoral action, public policy and health. Ottawa: Public Health Agency of Canada and Health Systems Knowledge Network; 2007.

7. Public Health Agency of Canada. Canada's response to WHO Commission on Social Determinants of Health. Ottawa: Public Health Agency of Canada; 2007.

8. Teeple, G. Globalization and the decline of social reform: Into the twenty-first century. Aurora, Ontario: Garamond Press; 2000.

9. Coburn, D. Beyond the income inequality hypothesis: Globalization, neo-liberalism, and health inequalities. Soc Sci Med. 2004;58:41–56.

10. Esping-Andersen, G. The three worlds of welfare capitalism. Princeton, NJ: Princeton University Press; 1990.

11. Esping-Andersen, G. Social foundations of post-industrial economies. New York: Oxford University Press; 1999.

12. Cohere, D. Health and health care: A political economy perspective. In: Raphael, D., Bryant, T., Rioux, M., editors. Staying alive: Critical perspectives on health, illness, and health care. Toronto: Canadian Scholars' Press; 2006. pp. 59–84.

13. Saint-Arnaud, S., Bernard, P. Convergence or resilience? A hierarchical cluster analysis of the welfare regimes in advanced countries. Curr Sociol. 2003;51(5):499–527.

14. Bernard, P., Saint-Arnaud, S. More of the same: The position of the four largest Canadian provinces in the world of welfare regimes. Ottawa: Canadian Policy Research Networks; 2004.

15. Teeple, G. Foreword. In: Raphael, D., Bryant, T., Rioux, M., editors. Staying alive: critical perspectives on health, illness, and health care. Toronto: Canadian Scholars' Press: 2006. pp. 1–4.

16. Navarro, V., Shi, L. The political contest of social inequalities and health. Int J Health Services. 2001;31(1):1–21.

17. Langille, D. The political determinants of health. In: Raphael, D. editor. Social determinants of health: Canadian perspectives. Toronto: Canadian Scholars Press; 2004. pp. 283–96.

18. Raphael, D., Bryant, T. The State's role in promoting population health: Public health concerns in Canada, USA, UK, and Sweden. Health Policy. 2006;78:39–55.

19. Raphael D. Barriers to addressing the determinants of health: Public health units and poverty in Ontario, Canada. Health Promot Int. 2003;18:397–405.

20. Raphael, D. Health inequalities in Canada: Current discourses and implications for public health action. Crit Public Health. 2000;10(2):193–216.

21. Hofrichter, R. editor. Health and social justice: A reader on politics, ideology, and inequity in the distribution of disease. San Francisco, CA: Jossey Bass; 2003.

22. Raphael, D., Bryant, T. Maintaining population health in a period of welfare slate decline: Political economy as the missing dimension in health promotion theory and practice. Promot Educ. 2006;13(4):236–42.

23. Canadian Population Health Initiative. Select highlights on public views of the determinants of health. Ottawa: CPHI; 2004.

24. Eyles, J., Brimacombe, M., Chaulk, P., Stoddart, G., Pranger, T., Masse, O. What determines health? To where should we shift resources? Attitudes towards the determinants of health among multiple stakeholder groups in Prince Edward Island, Canada. Soc Sci Med. 2001;53(12):1611–19.

25. Paisley, J., Midgett, C., Brunetti, G., Tomasik, H. Heart health Hamilton-Wentworth survey: programming implications. Can J Public Policy. 2001;92:443–7.

26. Davey Smith, G., editor. Inequalities in health: Life course perspectives. Bristol UK: Policy Press; 2003.

27. Wilkinson, R., Marmot, M. Social determinants of health: The solid facts. Copenhagen, Denmark: World Health Organization, European Office; 2003.

28. Popay, J., Williams, G.H. editors. Researching the people's health. London, UK: Routledge; 1994.

29. Bryant, T. Role of knowledge in public health and health promotion policy change. Health Promot Int. 2002;17(1):89–98.

30. Bambra, C., Fox, D., Scott-Samuel, A. Towards a politics of health. Health Promot Int. 2005;20(2):187–93.

31. Alesina, A. Glaeser, E.L. Fighting poverty in the US and Europe: A world of difference. Toronto: Oxford University Press; 2004.

32. Canadian Public Health Association. CPHA policy statements. Ottawa: Canadian Public Health Association; 2001.

RECOMMENDED READINGS

1. Baum, F. (2008). The commission on the social determinants of health: Reinventing health promotion for the twenty-first century? *Critical Public Health, 18*(4), 457–466.

This article argues that the final report of the International Commission on the Social Determinants of Health and the reports of its knowledge hubs provide a strong basis for the regeneration of the health promotion movement.

2. Commission on the Social Determinants of Health (2008). *Closing the gap in a generation: Health equity through action on the social determinants of health.* Final Report of the Commission on Social Determinants of Health. Geneva: World Health Organization. Available at http://whqlibdoc.who.int/publications/2008/9789241563703_eng.pdf.

This report is the outcome of the Commission on the Social Determinants of Health and reflects a tremendous amount of effort to raise the issue of the social determinants of health.

3. Chronic Disease Alliance of Ontario. (2008). *Primer to action: Social determinants of health*, revised ed. Toronto, ON: Chronic Disease Alliance of Ontario. Available at www.ocdpa.on.ca/docs/PrimertoAction2-EN.pdf.

This is an electronic resource that helps people to understand and influence how the social determinants of health impact chronic disease. Set in an electronic, easy-to-read format, with hundreds of links and resources, it is a practical resource for busy health and community workers, activists in their capacity as staff, volunteers, or community members.

4. Eikemo, T. A., & Bambra, C. (2008). The welfare state: A glossary for public health. *Journal of Epidemiology and Community Health, 62*(1), 3–6.

Building upon interest the relation between different aspects of the welfare state and population health, this article explicitly defines key concepts in order to enable more researchers, practitioners, and policy-makers to engage with and contribute to this area of public health research.

5. Esping-Andersen, G. (1985). *Politics against markets: The social democratic road to power.* Princeton, NJ: Princeton University Press.

Esping-Andersen, G. (1990). *The three worlds of welfare capitalism.* Princeton, NJ: Princeton University Press.

Esping-Andersen, G. (1999). *Social foundations of post-industrial economies.* New York: Oxford University Press.

These three volumes provide key insights into different forms of the welfare state and how they affect health and quality of life. Canada is a liberal welfare state and provides the fewest benefits and supports to citizens. Esping-Andersen outlines how these differing forms of the welfare states came about and what can be done to improve them.

6. Hofrichter, R. (2003). The politics of health inequities: contested terrain. In *Health and social justice: A reader on ideology, and inequity in the distribution of disease*. San Francisco: Jossey Bass.

    Hofrichter's book outlines the political, economic, and ideological barriers to reducing health inequalities and building healthy public policy in the USA and Canada. His chapter "The politics of health inequities: contested terrain" outlines why it is so difficult to implement policies that support health and quality of life.

7. Navarro, V. (Ed.). (2002). *The political economy of social inequalities: Consequences for health and quality of life*. Amityville, NY: Baywood Press.

    Navarro, V. (2007). *Neo-liberalism, globalization and inequalities: Consequences for health and quality of life*. Amityville, New York: Baywood Publishing Company, Inc.

    Navarro, V., & Muntaner, C. (Eds.). (2004). *Political and economic determinants of population health and well-being: Controversies and developments*. Amityville NY: Baywood Press.

    These three collections of papers explicitly consider how ideology and politics influence the social determinants of health. The importance of the welfare state for health is clearly demonstrated.

8. Raphael, D. (2007). The future of the Canadian welfare state. In D. Raphael (ed.), *Poverty and policy in Canada: Implications for health and quality of life*. Toronto, ON: Canadian Scholars' Press Inc.

    This chapter places the Canadian scene in a welfare state perspective. Being a liberal welfare state raises many barriers to improving health and quality of life through public policy action in Canada.

9. Raphael, D. (2008). Grasping at straws: A recent history of health promotion in Canada. *Critical Public Health, 18*, 483–495.

    This article outlines why health promotion concepts and approaches have proven so difficult to implement in Canada. Despite the rhetoric, Canada's health promotion approach has always stressed lifestyle and behavioural approaches at the expense of influencing structural aspects of society and its institutions.

10. Raphael, D., and Curry-Stevens, S. (2008). Surmounting the barriers: What will it take to prioritize the social determinants of health? In D. Raphael (ed.), *Social determinants of health: Canadian perspectives*, 2nd ed. Toronto, ON: Canadian Scholars' Press Inc.

    This chapter suggests avenues of activity to improve health and quality of life as well as discussing barriers to such activities.

RECOMMENDED WEBSITES

1. Canadian Centre for Policy Alternatives—www.policyalternatives.ca

   The centre monitors developments and promotes research on economic and social issues facing Canada. It provides alternatives to the views of business research institutes and many government agencies by publishing research reports, sponsoring conferences, organizing briefings, and providing informed comment on the issues of the day from a non-partisan perspective.

2. Caledon Institute of Social Policy—www.caledoninst.org

   The Caledon Institute provides research and analysis; seeks to inform and influence public opinion and to foster public discussion on poverty and social policy; and develops and promotes concrete, practicable proposals for the reform of social programs at all levels of government and of social benefits provided by employers and the voluntary sector.

3. Campaign 2000—www.campaign2000.ca

   This site is an excellent source of child-centred information on federal and provincial budgets, political debates, and demographic reports. The campaign began shortly after the all-party motion to end child poverty. When it appeared that little progress was underway, a group of non-governmental organizations and associated researchers came together to influence public policy and to strengthen family life in Canada, with the goal of making sure that no Canadian child is raised in poverty. The deadline has come and gone, with one-sixth of Canadian children living in poverty.

4. Canadian Council on Social Development (CCSD)—www.ccsd.ca

   The CCSD is a social policy and research organization focusing on social welfare and development issues of poverty, social inclusion, disability, cultural diversity, child well-being, employment, and housing. It provides statistics and reports on the state of poverty and income inequality in Canada and policy options for improving the health and well-being of Canadians.

5. Canadian Policy Research Networks—www.cprn.org

   This is the website of a non-profit policy think tank that undertakes research to guide decision-makers as they craft social and economic policy. It aims to advise Canada's leaders on the issues of our times and the policy options to move Canada forward. Its mission is to create knowledge and lead public dialogue and discussion on social and economic issues important to the well-being of all Canadians.

6. Centre for Social Justice—www.socialjustice.org

   The Centre for Social Justice conducts research, education, and advocacy in a bid to narrow gaps in income, wealth, and power, and enhance peace and human security. It brings together people from universities and unions, faith groups, and community organizations in the pursuit of greater equality and democracy.

7. Conference Board of Canada—www.conferenceboard.ca

   The mission of the Conference Board is to build leadership capacity for a better Canada by creating and sharing insights on economic trends, public policy, and organizational performance. Its reports *Defining the Canadian Advantage* and *Performance and Potential: The World and Canada* compare Canada to other nations on numerous quality of life indicators.

8. Federation of Canadian Municipalities (FCM)—www.fcm.ca

   FCM has been the national voice of municipal government since 1901. It represents the interests of municipalities on policy and program matters that fall within the federal jurisdiction. Members include Canada's largest cities, small urban and rural communities, and 18 provincial and territorial municipal associations.

9. Canada Without Poverty—www.cwp-csp.ca

   Formerly the National Anti-Poverty Organization, Canada without Poverty is a non-profit organization representing 4.7 million Canadians currently living in poverty. Its mandate is to eradicate poverty in this country. Its 19-member board is made up of people who currently live in poverty or who have lived in poverty at some time in their lives, and its membership is made up of low-income individuals, organizations that provide direct and indirect services to the poor, and other concerned Canadians.

10. National Council of Welfare (NCW)—www.ncwcnbes.net

   The NCW advises the Canadian government on matters related to social welfare and the needs of low-income Canadians. It publishes several reports each year on poverty and social policy issues. It also provides critical analyses of measurement issues and how these instruments compare to the amount of monies provided to people who are on social assistance or to the working poor.

Conclusion

CHAPTER 24

Can Increasing Concern with Quality of Life Encourage Health Promoting Public Policy?

Dennis Raphael

INTRODUCTION

Quality of life continues to be a concept with the potential to shape public policymaking in the service of health in Canada. However, like many other health-related concepts that move beyond narrow biomedical and behavioural risk concerns, it is not a front-and-centre issue for most Canadians. Much of this has to do with the continuing dominance of medical research and the narrow coverage of health issues by the media. When faced with an ongoing deluge from health authorities, governmental agencies, and the media as to the importance of medical and health care "breakthroughs" and the "holy trinity of risk" (Nettleton, 1997)—tobacco use, physical inactivity, and poor diet—there is little space for a quality of life agenda supported by healthy public policy.

In the academic sphere the great majority of "quality of life" research continues to be focused on very narrow outcomes associated with medical treatments of diseases and illnesses. For example, the academic journal *Quality of Life Research* defines itself as "An international journal of quality of life aspects of treatment, care and rehabilitation." And the media certainly reinforces this perspective through its limited reporting of health issues. For the most part the media limits its reporting to health care system issues such as funding and waiting times for treatment, research studies on outcomes of medical treatments, and often contradictory findings from studies that focus on risk factors for various diseases (Gasher et al., 2007; Hayes et al., 2007). Significant exertion will therefore be required to raise a broader-based vision of quality of life and its relation to health. There are some developments, however, that can support these efforts, such as the various endeavours underway to improve quality of life in Canada. Some of these are based in local communities across Canada. There are also notable Pan-Canadian efforts to develop and document quality of life and related concepts by the Atkinson Foundation, Genuine Progress Indicators, the Canadian Policy Research Networks, the Conference Board of Canada, and the Federation of Canadian Municipalities.

International work by the United Nations' Human Development Program, UNICEF's Innocenti Research Centre, and the Organization for Economic Co-operation and Development (OECD) on numerous social and policy-related indicators places Canadian performance within a comparative perspective. Canada generally does not do well in such comparisons. These analyses help to highlight numerous quality of life issues and suggest the importance of addressing these.

The increasing recognition of the importance of the social determinants of health also provides a framework by which findings from these quality of life efforts can be related to health outcomes (Raphael, 2008b). Many of the indicators of quality of life are clearly related to the social determinants of health. Perhaps the quality of life concept might be a means of focusing attention upon the importance of creating and implementing public policies that can strengthen aspects of societal support for citizens that include social determinants of quality of life as well as of health.

CANADIAN DEVELOPMENTS IN CONCEPTUALIZING QUALITY OF LIFE AND RELATED CONCEPTS

Numerous Canadian initiatives are underway that consider quality of life issues. All of these focus on providing indicators of societal support of quality of life.

Quality of Life Research Unit

The Quality of Life Research Unit at the University of Toronto's model of quality of life and its related measurement instruments that assess the domains of *Being*, *Belonging*, and *Becoming* continue to be applied in various settings (Quality of Life Research Unit, 2009). These activities include applications of the various measurement instruments for assessing individual quality of life; the community approach applying a community quality of life manual; and the participatory policy approach. The quality of life model has also been applied to organize and define how the experience of material and social deprivation (i.e. living in poverty) influences health and quality of life (Raphael, 2007c).

Neighbourhood Quality of Life Indicators Project, Saskatoon

An example of a community-based effort is that of the Development of Neighbourhood Quality of Life Indicators Project in Saskatoon. The domains chosen for this work are housing, health, employment and income, crime and safety, education, land-use and environment, social environment and services, and community participation. The purpose of the project is to provide information that governmental authorities can use to improve quality of life.

The project is participatory in that it has acted to engage the community in developing strategies and setting action priorities. The project, its processes, and its outcomes served as a basis for a special issue of *Social Indicators Research* (2008, vol. 85, no. 1). This issue contains 10 articles related to the quality of life aspect of the project (Kitchen & Muhajarine, 2008).

Atkinson Foundation's Canadian Index of Well-being

In terms of indicator projects, the Atkinson Foundation's Canadian Index of Well-being identifies the following domains: healthy population, community vitality, time use, educated populace, ecosystems health, arts and culture, civic engagement, and living standards.

The index has undergone an extensive development and validation process and has been released (Atkinson Foundation, 2009).

Canadian Policy Research Networks Quality of Life Project

The Canadian Policy Research Networks' model of quality of life has seen application in *Quality of Life in Canada: A Citizen's Report Card* (Canadian Policy Research Networks, 2002). The model includes 40 indicators organized around nine themes: economy/employment, government, democracy, health, environment, education, social conditions, personal well-being, and community (Michalski, 2001).

The findings presented in the *Report Card* were generally negative. Voter turnout is declining; Canadians believe discrimination is increasing and that access to health care can be improved; and air quality is declining and Canadians are concerned about water quality. Many Canadians live in poverty and social assistance lags below low-income cut-offs, although the number of Canadians using food banks has stabilized. Affordable housing is becoming less available. Trust in government is increasing, but faith in the electoral process is declining.

Conference Board of Canada Performance Project

The Conference Board of Canada's *How Canada Performs: A Report Card on Canada* describes the status of a variety of indicators in the areas of economy, innovation, health, environment, education and skills, and society (Conference Board of Canada, 2008). The reports compare Canada with other wealthy industrialized nations. In the most recent report Canada was awarded the following grades: economy (B), innovation (D), environment (C), education and skills (B), health (B), and society (B). The report comments: "While a 'B' grade in four categories may appear good enough, Canada's performance on many indicators is slipping, causing it to fall behind countries that are its peers, partners and competitors." The report also comments: "While Canada enjoys a standard of living that is the envy of many countries, our ranking dropped from 4th in 1990 to 9th now" (Conference Board of Canada, 2008).

Genuine Progress Indicator, Atlantic

Genuine Progress Indicator (GPI) Atlantic is a non-profit research and education organization that is creating a Genuine Progress Index for Nova Scotia (Genuine Progress Atlantic, 2009). Over the past 10 years, GPI Atlantic has produced more than 80 carefully researched reports on topics within the six main categories that make up the Genuine Progress Index: living standards, population health, time use, community vitality, education, and environmental quality. Reports such as *Financial Security and Debt in Atlantic Canada, Economic Security in Nova Scotia,* and *The Gender Wage Gap in New Brunswick* provide real insights into the nature of quality of life and its importance for public policymaking.

Federation of Canadian Municipalities' Quality of Life Reporting System

The Federation of Canadian Municipalities' (FCM's) Quality of Life Reporting System provides numerous indicators in the broad domains of demographic and background information, affordable and appropriate housing, civic engagement, community and social infrastructure, education, employment, local economy, natural environment, personal and community health, personal financial security, and personal safety (Federation of Canadian Municipalities, 1999).

The FCM has issued a number of quality of life reports that address important urban quality of life issues. Some of these are sharply critical of governments' efforts to support quality of life in Canada cities. The titles of and excerpts from these reports give a sense of their content and tone:

2009—IMMIGRATION AND DIVERSITY IN CANADIAN CITIES AND COMMUNITIES (FEDERATION OF CANADIAN MUNICIPALITIES, 2009)

> Recent immigrants are suffering from high rates of under-employment and poverty. This has significant implications for municipal governments, as they struggle to provide

adequate affordable housing, emergency shelters, social assistance and public health services to newcomers.

2008—TRENDS AND ISSUES IN AFFORDABLE HOUSING AND HOMELESSNESS (FEDERATION OF CANADIAN MUNICIPALITIES, 2008)

The estimated 150,000 to 200,000 homeless people in Canada
are the visible tip of a much larger population of financially
marginal individuals and households that are at risk of ending
up on the street. According to some estimates, some 700,000
households nation-wide are spending more than half of their
income on shelter, leaving them at considerable risk of homelessness, with some 600,000 to 650,000 people, many of them
children, living in inadequate or sub-standard housing.

2004—INCOMES, SHELTER AND NECESSITIES (FEDERATION OF CANADIAN MUNICIPALITIES, 2004)

This report points to the severe lack of affordable housing as
a prime cause of economic hardship among children, single-
parent families and seniors living in the 20 QOLRS communities. The shortage of affordable housing is among the most
pressing issues facing municipalities. It means too many people, particularly single-parent families, living in temporary
shelter or crowed into sub-standard and sometimes unsafe
housing. It also means more people living on the streets and
straining the ability of social service agencies to help them.

2003—FALLING BEHIND: OUR GROWING INCOME GAP (FEDERATION OF CANADIAN MUNICIPALITIES, 2003)

The three cities in this study are very different. Saskatoon,
Calgary, and Toronto are significantly different in their
physical size, composition, economy, population size and
composition. Therefore, commonalities were initially difficult to identify. However, upon completion of the study, it
is clear that the cities share a common challenge in terms of
growing income disparities and their impact. This suggests

that the income gap and income polarization is greater than an isolated big-city problem.

The data in the FCM reports—and most others—document a growing gap in income among urban residents, an increasing lack of affordable housing, and an increasing gap between minimum wages, social assistance rates, and housing rental rates. It is rather striking that there seems to be so much overlap between the indicators coming from these projects and the social determinants of health of Aboriginal status, early life, education, employment and working conditions, food security, gender, health care services, housing, income and its distribution, the social safety net, social exclusion, unemployment, and employment security. Indeed, I frequently cite findings from these quality of life and related projects in support of the need for public policy action to strengthen the social determinants of health.

INTERNATIONAL DEVELOPMENTS IN CONCEPTUALIZING QUALITY OF LIFE AND RELATED CONCEPTS

A variety of international indicator projects place Canada's quality of life in comparative perspective. Generally, Canada's welfare state—an important contributor to quality of life—is undeveloped as compared to that of other wealthy developed nations.

United Nations' Human Development Report

For many years the United Nations' Human Development Program has been documenting how nations perform on a variety of indices that are clearly related to quality of life (United Nations Human Development Program, 2009). The Human Development Index is a composite measure of three dimensions of human development: life expectancy, adult literacy and enrolment at the primary, secondary, and tertiary level of education, and income (per capita gross domestic product [GDP]). In 2007, Canada did rather well coming in fourth among the world's nations. Canada ranked eleventh in life expectancy, fifth in education, and 15th in income (United Nations Human Development Program, 2009).

However, Canada did less well in the Human Poverty Index, achieving a rank of twelfth, and on the Gender Equity Measure, achieved a rank of fourth. The report provides hundreds of indicators on which Canada's performance can be compared with other nations.

Innocenti Centre Report Cards on Children's Health and Well-being

The series of report cards issued by the Innocenti Centre of UNICEF on children's health and well-being provides a more troubling picture (UNICEF, 2009). In 2005, Canada's infant mortality rate was compared to that of 30 wealthy developed nations of the OECD (Innocenti Research Centre, 2007). Canada's rate gave it a relative ranking of 24th of 30 nations. Canada's low birth-weight rate provided a somewhat better ranking of ninth of 30 nations.

During the period 1991–1995, Canadian children died from injuries at levels that gave it a ranking of 18th of 26 wealthy industrialized nations for which data were available (Innocenti Research Centre, 2001a). Canada's teenage pregnancy rate during the 1990s provided a rank of 21st of 28 nations (Innocenti Research Centre, 2001b).

Further analyses of the range of health determinants and Canada's place among developed nations can be seen in a report by the Innocenti Research Centre entitled *An Overview of Child Well-being in Rich Countries: A Comprehensive Assessment of the Lives and Well-Being of Children and Adolescents in the Economically Advanced Nations* (Innocenti Research Centre, 2007). Twenty-one OECD nations were included in the analysis. Overall, Canada ranked 12th of 21 nations. Canada's thematic rankings were as follows: material well-being, sixth of 21; health and safety, 13th of 21; educational well-being, second of 18; family and peer relationships, 18th of 21; behaviours and risks, 17th of 21; and subjective well-being, 15th of 21.

Society at a Glance, Education at a Glance, Health at a Glance

The series of reports on various societal indicators issued by the OECD, specifically *Society at a Glance, Health at a Glance,* and *Education at a Glance,* place Canadian public policy within a comparative perspective (Organisation for Economic Co-operation and Development, 2009). To summarize briefly, Canada's scores on a variety of indicators of providing citizens with economic security are rather low in a comparative perspective.

One important indicator of economic security provision is extent of government transfers to households (Organization for Economic Co-operation and Development, 2008). Transfers refer to governments taking fiscal resources that are generated by the economy and distributing them to the population as services, monetary supports, or investments in social infrastructure. Such infrastructure includes education, employment training, social assistance or welfare payments, family supports, pensions, health and social services, and other benefits.

Canada ranks 18th of 24 wealthy industrialized nations (for which 2003 data are available) and spent 19.6% of GDP on public expenditures (Organization for Economic Co-operation and Development, 2008). How does spending translate into specific policy areas? Canada is among the highest spenders on health care (6.8% of GDP), exceeded by only a few nations: Germany, the USA, France, Belgium, Iceland, and Sweden. It is in the other areas of benefits and supports to citizens that Canada reveals itself as a frugal public spender.

Canada ranks very low on income supports to the working-age population and social services (Organization for Economic Co-operation and Development, 2008). In 2001, Canada spent just 2.8% of GDP in income supports to the working-age population (rank 27th of 30) and 2.2% on social services (rank eighth of 30). Active labour policy refers to the extent that governments support training and other policies that foster employment and reduces unemployment. In 2003, Canada allocated 0.4% of GDP to such policies, which provides Canada with a ranking of 19th of 29 wealthy industrialized nations for which data were available. Further presentation of these types of data is available (Raphael, 2007a).

CANADIAN DEVELOPMENTS IN THE SOCIAL DETERMINANTS OF HEALTH AREA

The Toronto Charter on the Social Determinants of Health outlines the importance of addressing the living conditions to which Canadians are exposed. There have been some notable recent developments in the social determinants of health field in Canada. This has been assisted by the World Health Organization's International Commission on the Social Determinants of Health issuing its final report (World Health Organization, 2008). Two of the Commission's knowledge networks (globalization and health and early childhood development) were centred in Canada, and another (workplace health) had significant Canadian representation. These networks' final reports are available (World Health Organization, 2009). In addition, the Canadian Senate's Subcommittee on Population Health has undertaken a review of the social determinants of health (Canadian Senate, 2007).

Within Canada, a few Canadian health units have distinguished themselves by their work in raising the importance of the social determinants of health (Raphael, 2007b). The Public Health Agency of Canada has established a National Coordinating Centre for the Determinants of Health at St. Francis Xavier University in Nova Scotia (Government of Canada, 2004).

In addition, there is clear evidence that those working in specific social determinants of health concept areas such as employment security and working conditions, early childhood education and care, housing, income, food security, health and social services, and poverty reduction are becoming more aware of how their issues impact health (Raphael, 2008b). Non-governmental agencies such as United Ways across Canada and the United Nations Association of Canada have drawn upon the social determinants of health concept to advance their work (United Nations Association of Canada, 2006; United Way of Greater Toronto & Canadian Council on Social Development, 2002; United Way of Ottawa, 2003; United Way of Winnipeg, 2003).

IMPLICATIONS FOR HEALTH PROMOTION

While it is clear that there are numerous quality of life activities occurring, there is little evidence that these activities—or those associated with the social determinants of health concept—have significantly contributed to Canadian public policy advances in the service of health (Raphael, Curry-Stevens, & Bryant, 2008). This is the case despite evidence that Canadian performance on these indicators leaves much to be desired. When governments do produce health-enhancing public policies such as new housing programs or enhanced early-childhood education programs—and there is less and less of that happening these days—it is difficult to discern health considerations as having entered into their decisions. This has not been the case elsewhere, where social determinants of health concepts have been actively incorporated into the making of public policy (Mackenbach & Bakker, 2002).

Baum has suggested that the final report from the International Commission on the Social Determinants of Health, *Achieving Equity in a Generation*, can serve as stimulus for citizen action through a health-promotion perspective (Baum, 2008). Baum points out that the report identifies three key issues, all of which are consistent with a health-promotion approach. These are the importance of: (i) improving the daily living conditions in which people are born, grow, live, work, and age; (ii) tackling the inequitable distribution of power, money, and resources—the structural drivers of daily living conditions—globally, nationally, and locally; and (iii) measuring and understanding the problem of health inequities and assessing the impact of action.

However, health promotion may be becoming ill-equipped to handle this task. There is increasing concern about its future in Canada (Raphael, 2008a). Much of this is related to weakening governmental and agency commitment to the principles of health promotion—equity, citizen engagement, and addressing the prerequisites of health—as outlined in the Ottawa Charter for Health Promotion. There are various reasons why this has occurred. The primary reason is that Canadian governments are becoming less active in improving the quality of numerous social determinants of health.

In the health field itself, health promotion has been weakened by two trends. The first is an increasing emphasis on behavioural risk factors or healthy lifestyles by governments, health agencies, and the media (Raphael, 2008a). The second is increasing academic acceptance of the population health position with its emphasis on expert-driven epidemiological approaches to understanding health as opposed to a citizen-based social movement that strives to attain control over the determinants of health (Raphael & Bryant, 2002). Between these approaches there is little room for a citizen-focused health promotion strategy focused on creating public policy that supports improved quality of life. There is a need for those committed to health promotion principles and activities to take advantage of the increasing activities and growing concern with quality of life and the social determinants to reinvent health promotion (O'Neill et al., 2007).

CONCLUSION

There is increasing evidence that the quality of life of Canadians is under threat. Numerous sets of indicators from varying sources confirm this impression. It has been argued that many of these quality of life indicators show similarities with what are now being termed the social determinants of health. Activity associated with the social determinants has been increasing with, however, rather little to show for it (Raphael, 2009).

Canadians require means of responding to these challenges and taking control over the determinants of both their quality of life and health. I propose that health promotion, as conceived by the Ottawa Charter for Health Promotion, continues to provide a means of accomplishing these goals.

As argued in the first chapter of this volume, health promotion is about engaging citizens in order to increase their control over the determinants of health. The best way to do this is to influence the development and implementation of health promoting public policy. To achieve this, health promotion will need to reinvent itself as a new social movement committed to improving quality of life and the social determinants of health.

It is altogether fitting that this be so, as many health promotion concepts originated in Canada. But there are barriers to a re-emergence of health promotion. These barriers include a weakening commitment on the part of governments to address the determinants of both quality of life and health, and a continued weakened health sector commitment to health promotion principles.

Baum has forcefully argued that the work of the International Commission on the Social Determinants of health can serve to re-energize the health promotion movement (Baum, 2008). There clearly is a close association between quality of life, the social determinants of health, and the possibilities offered by the principles and values of health promotion. Considering the evidence concerning the quality of life situation in Canada, let us hope that the emergence of a new health promotion movement can occur.

REFERENCES

Atkinson Foundation. (2009). *Canadian index of wellness*. Retrieved April 15, 2009, from http://www.atkinsonfoundation.ca/ciw

Baum, F. (2008). The Commission on the Social Determinants of Health: Reinventing health promotion for the twenty-first century? *Critical Public Health*, 18(4), 457–466.

Canadian Policy Research Networks. (2002). *Quality of life in Canada: A citizens' report card*. Retrieved July 9, 2009, from http://www.cprn.org/doc.cfm?doc=44&l=en

Canadian Senate. (2007). *Sub-committee on population health*. Retrieved September 5, 2007, from http://tinyurl.com/ypwhhq

Conference Board of Canada. (2008). *How Canada performs: A report card on Canada*. Retrieved April 15, 2009, from http://www.conferenceboard.ca/HCP/default.aspx

Federation of Canadian Municipalities. (1999). *Quality of life reporting system: Quality of life in Canadian communities*. Ottawa, ON: Federation of Canadian Municipalities (FCM).

Federation of Canadian Municipalities. (2003). *Falling behind: our growing income gap*. Retrieved July 9, 2004, from http://www.fcm.ca/CMFiles/falling1v-fr-3272008-7169.pdf

Federation of Canadian Municipalities. (2004). *Income, shelter and necessities*. Ottawa, ON: Federation of Canadian Municipalities.

Federation of Canadian Municipalities. (2008). *Trends and issues in affordable housing and homelessness*. Ottawa, ON: Federation of Canadian Municipalities.

Federation of Canadian Municipalities. (2009). *Immigration and diversity in Canadian cities and communities*. Ottawa, ON: Federation of Canadian Municipalities.

Gasher, M., Hayes, M., Ross, I., & Dunn, J. (2007). Spreading the news: Social determinants of health reportage in Canadian daily newspapers. *Canadian Journal of Communication*, 32(3), 557–574.

Genuine Progress Atlantic. (2009). *Genuine progress index for Atlantic Canada*. Retrieved April 15, 2009, from http://www.gpiatlantic.org

Government of Canada. (2004). *Government of Canada announces national collaborating centre for determinants of health.* Retrieved September 14, 2005, from http://www.phac-aspc.gc.ca/media/nr-rp/2004/2004_02_e.html

Hayes, M., Ross, I. E., Gasher, M., Gustein, D., Dunn, J. R., & Hackett, R. A. (2007). Telling stories: News media, health literacy and public policy in Canada. *Social Science and Medicine, 64*(9), 1842–1852.

Innocenti Research Centre. (2001a). *A league table of child deaths by injury in rich nations.* Florence: Innocenti Research Centre.

Innocenti Research Centre. (2001b). *A league table of teenage births in rich nations.* Florence: Innocenti Research Centre.

Innocenti Research Centre. (2007). *An overview of child well-being in rich countries: a comprehensive assessment of the lives and well-being of children and adolescents in the economically advanced nations.* Florence: Innocenti Research Centre.

Kitchen, P., & Muhajarine, N. (2008). Quality of life research: New challenges and new opportunities. *Social Indicators Research, 85*(1), 1–4.

Mackenbach, J., & Bakker, M. (Eds.). (2002). *Reducing inequalities in health: A European perspective.* London, UK: Routledge.

Michalski, J. H. (2001). *Asking citizens what matters for quality of life in Canada: Results of CPRN's public dialogue process.* Ottawa, ON: Canadian Policy Research Networks.

Nettleton, S. (1997). Surveillance, health promotion and the formation of a risk identity. In M. Sidell, L. Jones, J. Katz, & A. Peberdy (Eds.), *Debates and Dilemmas in Promoting Health* (pp. 314–324). London, UK: Open University Press.

O'Neill, M., Pederson, A., Dupéré, S., & Rootman, I. (Eds.). (2007). *Health promotion in Canada: Critical perspectives.* Toronto, ON: Canadian Scholars' Press Inc.

Organisation for Economic Co-operation and Development. (2009). *Publications.* Retrieved April 15, 2009, from http://www.oecd.org/publications

Organization for Economic Co-operation and Development. (2008). *Society at a glance: OECD social indicators,* 2008 ed. Paris, France.

Quality of Life Research Unit. (2009). *Quality of life.* Retrieved April 15, 2009, from http://www.utoronto.ca/qol

Raphael, D. (2007a). Canadian public policy and poverty in international perspective. In D. Raphael (Ed.), *Poverty and policy in Canada: Implications for health and quality of life* (pp. 335–364). Toronto, ON: Canadian Scholars' Press Inc.

Raphael, D. (2007b). *Poverty and policy in Canada: Implications for health and quality of life.* Toronto, ON: Canadian Scholars' Press Inc.

Raphael, D. (2007c). Poverty and quality of life. In D. Raphael (Ed.), *Poverty and policy in Canada: Implications for health and quality of life* (pp. 269–302). Toronto, ON: Canadian Scholars' Press Inc.

Raphael, D. (2008a). Grasping at straws: A recent history of health promotion in Canada. *Critical Public Health, 18*(4), 483–495.

Raphael, D. (Ed.). (2008b). *Social determinants of health: Canadian perspectives,* 2nd ed. Toronto, ON: Canadian Scholars' Press Inc.

Raphael, D. (2009). Escaping from the phantom zone: social determinants of health, public health units and public policy in Canada. *Health Promotion International, 24*(2), 193–198.

Raphael, D., & Bryant, T. (2002). The limitations of population health as a model for a new public health. *Health Promotion International, 17,* 189–199.

Raphael, D., Curry-Stevens, A., & Bryant, T. (2008). Barriers to addressing the social determinants of health: Insights from the Canadian experience. *Health Policy, 88,* 222–235.

UNICEF. (2009). *Innocenti Research Centre.* Retrieved April 15, 2009, from http://www.unicef-irc.org

United Nations Association of Canada. (2006). *Healthy children, healthy communities.* Retrieved June 22, 2006, from http://www.unac.org/hchc/en/index.php

United Nations Human Development Program. (2008). *Human development report 2007/2008. Fighting climate change: human solidarity in a divided world.* New York: United Nations Human Development Program.

United Nations Human Development Program. (2009). *Human development reports.* Retrieved April 15, 2009, from http://hdr.undp.org/en

United Way of Greater Toronto, & Canadian Council on Social Development. (2002). *A decade of decline: Poverty and income inequality in the City of Toronto in the 1990s.* Toronto, ON: Canadian Council on Social Development and United Way of Greater Toronto.

United Way of Ottawa. (2003). *Environmental scan.* Ottawa, ON: United Way of Ottawa.

United Way of Winnipeg. (2003). *2003 Environmental scan and Winnipeg census data.* Winnipeg, MB: United Way of Winnipeg.

World Health Organization. (2008). *Closing the gap in a generation: Health equity through action on the social determinants of health.* Geneva: World Health Organization.

World Health Organization. (2009). *Social determinants of health.* Retrieved April 15, 2009, from http://www.who.int/social_determinants/en

Copyright Acknowledgments

Chapter 18

Clarke, W. (2002). *Economic gender equality indicators, 2000.* Ottawa: Status of Women Canada. Her Majesty the Queen in Right of Canada. All rights reserved. Copyright © Minister of Public Works and Government Services Canada, 2009. Reprinted with Permission.

Chapter 19

Raphael, D., Curry-Stevens, A., & Bryant, T. (2008). Barriers to addressing the social determinants of health: Insights from the Canadian experience. *Health Policy, 88,* 222-235. Copyright © Elsevier Inc. Reprinted with Permission.

Chapter 20

Raphael, D., Labonte, R., Colman, R., Hayward, K., Torgerson, R., Macdonald J. (2006) Income and Health in Canada: Research Gaps and Future Opportunities. *Canadian Journal of Public Health, 97* (Supplement 3), Sept–Oct 2006, S16-S23. Copyright © Canadian Public Health Association. Reprinted with permission.

Chapter 21

Bryant, T., Raphael, D., & Travers, R. (2007). Identifying and strengthening the structural roots of urban health: Participatory policy research and the Canadian urban health agenda. *Promotion and Education, 2007, 14* (1), 2007, 6-11. Copyright © Sage Publications. Reprinted with permission.

Chapter 22

Raphael, D. (2008). Getting serious about addressing the social determinants of health: New directions for public health researchers and workers. *Promotion and Education, 15* (3): 15-20.Copyright © Sage Publications. Reprinted with permission.